THE
9-INCH
"DIET"

THE 9-INCH "DIET"

EXPOSING THE BIG CONSPIRACY IN AMERICA

BY ALEX BOGUSKY

WITH A LITTLE HELP FROM CHUCK PORTER

 powerHouse Books Brooklyn, NY

ACKNOWLEDGEMENTS

Chuck and I received so much help and love from people that we could probably go on thanking folks for several pages, but we'll keep it short. Thanks to Robin Fitzgerald and David Steinke, who broke the ice on this project with Chuck and me. Thanks to Mike Kohlbecker for jumping in on the design and art direction down the home stretch. Wouldn't have gotten finished without him.

Thanks to Jason Ambrose, John Broe, Catherine Christiansen, Meghan DeBruler, Cathy Dickinson, Andrew Dixon, Louise Doherty, Ryan Eckert, Emily Einheit, Colby Graff, Charlyn Hare, Jake Harvey, Jessica Hoffman, Mel Kreilein, Eric Lear, David Littlejohn, Brian McMillen, Joshua Merced, Marco Merced, Crystal Newberry, Kari Niessink, Peter Nolan, China Paradelo, Wayne Porter, Brian Rekasis, Renée Schoichit, Amanda Schultz, and Anh Truong, from production to proofreading.

And thanks to Daniel Power, Craig Cohen, and Kiki Bauer from powerHouse Books for keeping a fire lit under our tushies for the last couple of years.

Finally, I'd like to thank my wife, Ana, who is my gravity and without whom I would just float away.

CONTENTS

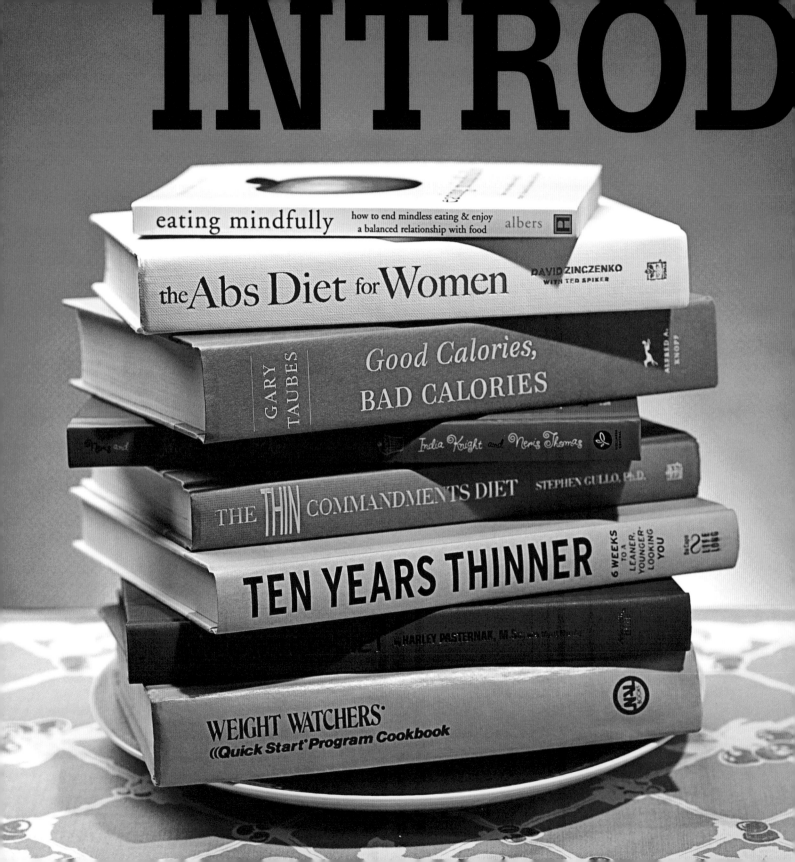

UCTION

"DIET"?

Some of you may have already noticed that the word "diet" on the cover of this book is in quotes. "Why is that?" you might wonder. "Is this not truly a diet book?" you ask. Very good questions, and I'm so glad you picked up on that.

The "why" is simple. It is my opinion that diets don't work.

There, I said it. Pretty bold words for a first-time "diet" book writer, but if you're looking for a traditional diet book, now would be a good time to close this one up and move on.

Good, they're gone. I knew they weren't in it for the long haul. For those of you still reading, let me clarify. I'm not saying that a person cannot lose weight on a special diet. In fact (insert sarcastic tone here), a whopping one in twenty diets works. One in twenty! Pretty dismal results. The truth is, most of us have spent some time riding the weight yo-yo. But very few have experienced a long-term change in weight. Soon the weight comes back on, and then it's time for a new fad diet and a new diet book to start

Hershey's bar weighs 2 ounces, 297 calories.

the cycle all over again. The diets aren't all bad. I'm certainly not here to defend them, but in a perfect world, they probably would work. But that's just the problem. The world we live in is not perfect. It's not logical. And maybe I'm just being dramatic, but the world of food is even less perfect than the world in general.

Culture informs behavior. We like to think we make rational decisions, but let me assure you we don't—not me, and not you either. I know it's hard to accept, but we live by the rules that our society lays out for us. We're all victims of popular culture.

1950

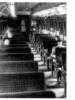

Average seat for train passengers measures 18 inches.

The trouble is that our popular food culture is one of large portions. Huge portions. Doled out in ways that make it truly impossible to identify how much we're eating. The rules have changed, and nobody told the players. So being successful on a diet in the face of all this prevailing cultural pressure is almost impossible. In fact, it's such a universal problem that, as a culture, we continue to churn through diets as fast as they can be invented. If diets actually worked, would we really need so many?

1952

Average woman's dress size: 8.

All of which leads us, conveniently, to the reason the word "diet" is on the cover. The word is powerful. It gets people to pick up books and buy them. But the definition has been distorted, and the hope I have is that the word can be fixed. That's the reason the word diet is in quotes. Because this is not really a diet book. This is a book designed to help you join and create a lifestyle and a subculture that enable you and your loved

1955

McDonald's fries weigh in at 2.4 ounces, 210 calories.

IF DIETS ACTUALLY WORKED, WOULD WE REALLY NEED SO MANY?

Average restaurant plate is 8 inches in diameter.

ones to eat less every day without the pressure of a special diet. Who knows, you and this book could start the swinging of the portion pendulum back in the other direction for a whole generation.

MOST DIETS DON'T CHANGE BEHAVIOR. LUCKILY, THAT'S WHAT I'M GOOD AT.

I must confess that I had no intention of ever being the writer of a diet book—or even a "diet" book, for that matter. It just happened. I'm neither a doctor nor a dietitian (but I doubt that anyone in either profession would find fault with what's in this book). No, my profession is, of all things, advertising. A fact that, according to statistics and market research, will make you suspicious of me right away. I like that. It seems to me you should start any book with some suspicion.

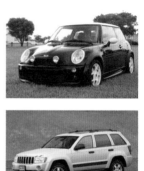

MINI VS. SUV

Advertising ranks just above used-car sales in terms of professions that engender public trust. This should not be a problem, though, because I'm considered an expert in what this book deals with—perception, popular culture, and the changing of behavior. In my years in the ad biz, I have worked on campaigns for dozens of clients, like Volkswagen, Coca-Cola, IKEA, Microsoft and Burger King. Yes, Burger King. Fast food. Like most of us I grew up on it and I still love it and eat it. This "diet" will work with any food because it's not about what. It's about how much.

1972

McDonald's introduces large fries (3.5 ounces).

1980

7-Eleven introduces the 32-ounce Big Gulp®, and it is the biggest cup on the market.

1981

Military MRE (Meals, Ready to Eat) are introduced. Size is 5 ounces.

And how to keep track of how much. Without scales and the stress of counting every calorie. A salad is nice. But a garbage-pail portion ain't doing anybody any good. I'm also considered largely responsible for an advertising campaign that turned around youth smoking. Researchers even determined that exposure to the truth® campaign was the largest, and arguably the only, reason for the reversal of teen tobacco consumption. It's even believed by many to be the most successful social marketing campaign of all time. Of course, the entire change in behavior happened because we were able to simply change kids' perception of their culture. Changes in perception of culture create changes in behavior. In my line of work, this is a fact we deal with every day.

It was exactly what we had to deal with when we introduced the MINI Cooper to America. We were about to launch the smallest car ever into the U.S. at a time when small-car sales were at the lowest in eight years and SUVs had all the momentum. The conventional thinking was that we needed to play up how big the MINI was inside. But we knew that to be successful, we needed to create momentum for the culture of small. So one of the first things we did was put up billboards in key buzz markets, showing the MINI and proclaiming, "The SUV backlash officially starts now." The funny thing is, there was no SUV backlash at the time. We made it up. We thought it was a good idea, but it hadn't happened. Well, soon it did. Six months after the campaign started, the *Atlanta Journal-Constitution* wrote an article outlining the three reasons for the SUV backlash. One of the reasons they cited was that billboard campaign.

1984

Bagels have 3-inch diameter, 140 calories.

1986

Standard TV has 27-inch screen.

1988

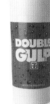

7-Eleven introduces the giant 64-ounce Double Gulp®, the biggest soft drink on the market.

1988

McDonald's introduces a 32-ounce "super-size" soda and "super-size" fries.

Cultural perceptions changed, and guess what else changed? Behavior. MINI sold out its entire year's inventory in nine months. But what might be even more amazing, and more telling, was that the entire small-car segment grew for the first time in eight years. So changing popular culture is what I do. To be successful at that, you usually have to try and step out of your everyday world and look back at it like an outsider. And sometimes what you see there is really weird.

THE LAKE HOUSE MYSTERY

This book came about because of one event. I bought a lake house. Now you might be thinking I needed the money to pay for the lake house and so I launched a scheme to write a diet book. To which I say, "Sorry, wrong." When are you going to stop jumping to conclusions? Anyway, it's a very quaint place that was built in the 1940s and, thank goodness for me and this story, the house had never been gutted or renovated. The whole place was original, including the kitchen. Well, it was a very exciting thing to have a lake house, and we couldn't wait to stock the place, so my wife and I made up a shopping list of basic things we would need for the kitchen, made our way to Target or somewhere, and loaded up on supplies. As soon as we got back to the house, we began putting everything away. But when we started putting the plates in the

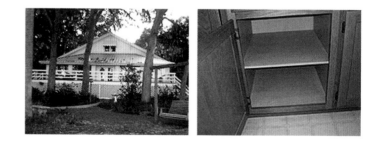

THE LAKE HOUSE (LEFT) AND ITS 60-YEAR-OLD CABINETS (RIGHT)

cupboards, they wouldn't fit. Literally. The cabinet doors could and would not close. Not by a mile. I tried the top shelf, the bottom shelf. I tried them on their sides, and I tried angling them. Wasn't going to happen.

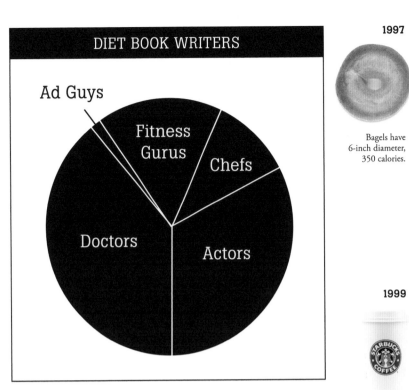

DIET BOOK WRITERS

Ad Guys

Fitness Gurus

Chefs

Doctors

Actors

"What kind of idiot builds a cupboard that doesn't hold a normal plate?" I thought. See, I was still playing by the rules of the existing food culture, and this situation simply made no sense. So I did what I'm trained to do. I stood back and removed all of my preconceived notions. I do this by scratching the top of my head. Soon I scratched myself to an epiphany. I realized that there is no "idiot" who would build a cupboard too small to hold a "normal" plate. What had happened is that "normal" must have changed in the 60 years since that cupboard was built.

Suddenly my head was spinning with colliding ideas. As a guy pushing 40 I was dealing with pant sizes that kept getting bigger. I wasn't exactly heavy, but my shirt wasn't coming off a lot in public either. I was obviously eating too much because I was increasing in girth, but it didn't feel like it was too much. My perception was that I was having "normal" meals. I was confronted by this idea that generations before me (thinner generations)

1997

Bagels have 6-inch diameter, 350 calories.

1999

Starbucks introduces the 20-ounce "venti" size, and discontinues its 8-ounce cup.

2000

McDonald's "super-size" fries increase to 7 ounces (610 calories).

13

MOST PEOPLE WHO GREW UP IN THE 60S OR BEFORE HAVE ALREADY BEEN ON THIS DIET.

were having their "normal" meals on plates substantially smaller than mine. Damn, this was big news, and nobody knew the story. Hell, I didn't know the story yet. But I knew there were tremendous cultural ramifications of this missing-link plate. It could lead to a way to control portions (a very hot diet topic) and do it in a way that was effortless and "normal."

2002

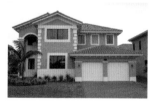

Average woman's dress size: 14.

"Oh, shit," I thought, "I'm about to write a diet book."

Here's some very good news to start the book off. Most people who grew up in the 60s or before have already been on this diet. And it worked. Of course, it wasn't called a diet then. It was just called breakfast, lunch, and dinner. Scrambled eggs. Spaghetti and meatballs. Baked ham, mashed potatoes, and green bean casserole. You passed the bowls to the left and filled up your plate (at the time, it measured about 8.5 inches). You didn't even think about it.

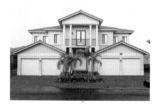

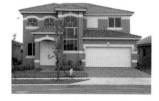

McMANSIONS

14

When your plate was clean (we'll cover this more later), you were done. Better than just done. Somehow, you were full and you were satisfied. Even after eating substantially less food than we do now.

Well, things have surely changed since then. Over the past 30 years, America has been suffering from a severe case of gigantism. In some ways, we've known it and even celebrated it. Cars have turned into station wagons, which have turned into vans, which have turned into two-ton SUVs. Family homes have turned into 20-room McMansions. And the food merchants have come up with a phrase that sums up the whole phenomenon, "super-size."

In this oversized new world, steaks are bigger, pizzas are bigger, sodas are bigger, and so are you.

You know it. We all know it. But the weird thing is that none of us is really aware of the changes because they have been too gradual to perceive. For every one thing you see that looks oversized, there are 10 oversized things that just look "normal."

Now while the media has made some noise about our food getting bigger and bigger, another thing has happened that you don't hear much about. The stuff our food sits on, and in, has gotten bigger as well. All of it. The plates have gotten bigger. So have the bowls and the cups and the glasses and even the knives and forks. Hell, even the tables have grown to fit all that bigness.

2003

Average restaurant plate is 12 inches.

2004

Theaters install 22-inch seats. Sport stadiums increase seat width from 19 inches to 24 inches.

2004

Standard TV has 40-inch to 60-inch screen.

15

If you're like most people, your "normal" (I may just put "normal" in quotes for the remainder of the book, since there is no such thing as "normal") everyday plates are about 40 percent bigger than they were in 1960. 40 percent. So you're automatically eating a lot more than people did then, and a lot more than you need to be eating now. The nine-inch "diet" is all about getting you back to "normal"-size nine-inch plates. And the results in reduced caloric intake—from that alone—are amazing.

PICK A DIET. ANY DIET.

Let's say you're already on some kind of "weight-loss program." Take your pick—Atkins, South Beach, Zone, Sugar Busters!, Weight Watchers, whatever. Or maybe you're about to start one. While I'm still skeptical of diets, I guarantee that the practical advice and cultural awareness you'll get from this book can make your diet more effective. In fact, it would be smart to get on the nine-inch "diet" before you start any other diet. That way, when you come off that radical weight-loss plan, your chances will be much higher than one in twenty of keeping the weight off. And it will be as easy and natural as sitting down to dinner.

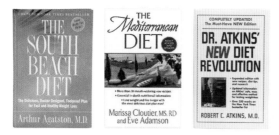

THE NINE-INCH "DIET" CAN MAKE THESE POPULAR WEIGHT-LOSS PROGRAMS MORE EFFECTIVE

Now some of you may assume you've already read enough to know all you need to know. Get some smaller plates, badda-boom-badda-bing, and you're golden. For you I should have written

THERE IS A TWISTED CONSPIRACY THAT IS MAKING OUR COUNTRY FAT.

a pamphlet. The bad news is, you'll be missing the point of the whole book. Since this isn't a diet book and it is a "diet" book, you may just miss out on the revolution. And some laughs. Because there's much more going on here than just your buying some smaller plates. There is a twisted conspiracy that is making our country fat. And it won't change unless a lot of us start getting the word out. The nine-inch "diet" helps you see just how distorted your reality is. It shows you how to create a world for yourself in which you're eating in a different, healthier, more "normal" way. It begins to erase the 30 years of promotion and propaganda (started by the government, but we'll get to that later) that have resulted in a whole generation of overeaters. This book gives you dozens of really useful ideas that will help you change bad habits, grow good habits, and get to a healthier weight—permanently—without ever feeling like you're on a diet. These here pages are filled with so much practical advice that you'll end up wanting impractical advice. And, as you'll see, I threw some of that in, too. That's one of the benefits of being a "diet" book. No rules.

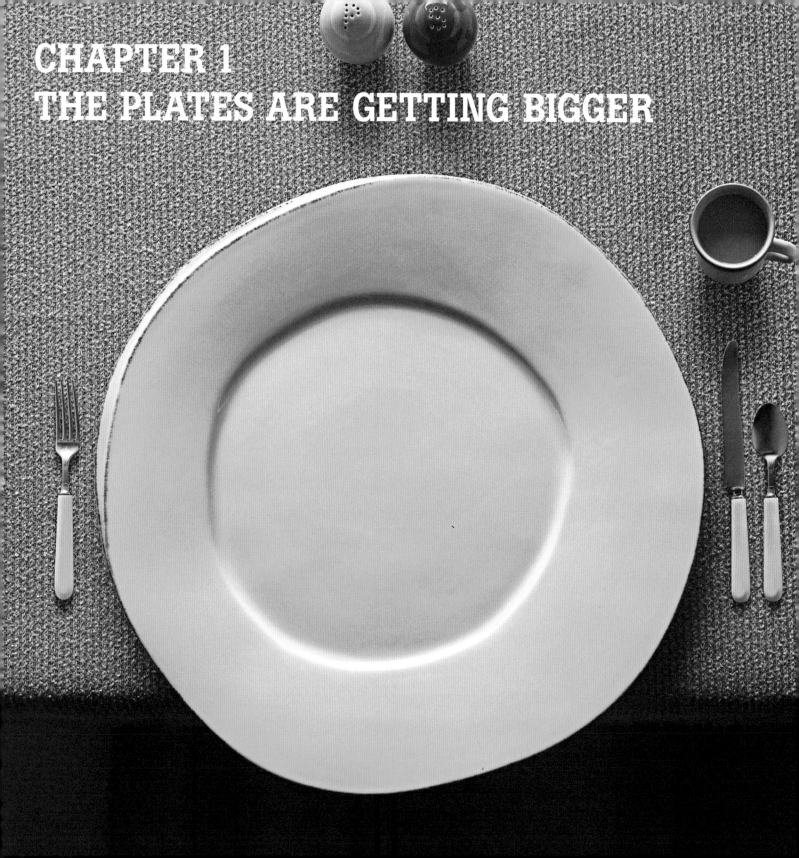

CHAPTER 1
THE PLATES ARE GETTING BIGGER

IF YOU'VE EVER THOUGHT THAT EVERYDAY PLATES SEEM BIGGER THAN THEY USED TO BE, YOU'RE NOT CRAZY. WELL, YOU MIGHT BE CRAZY, BUT YOU AREN'T MISTAKEN.

If, on the other hand, you find it hard to believe that plates have gone from an average of 8.5 inches to an average of 12 inches, then it's time for me to make my case.

It's a fact. The plates are getting bigger, and so are the glasses and everything else. And I'll bet if you think back, you've probably noticed it in one way or another. Maybe it happened to you one night when you were putting dishes away. In the incredible shrinking cupboard of any home built before 1981. Or, what about the last time you ate out? When you had to elbow water glasses and salt shakers out of the way so that a plate the size of a turkey platter could be lowered in front of you. Was it always like this? Not even close.

Through some sort of twisted cupboard evolution, dinner plates have become salad plates. And salad plates are now used for dessert. According to the American Institute for Cancer Research, the standard restaurant dinner plate has increased from 10 inches

to 12 inches just since 1970. And it's showing no signs of slowing.

The proof is pretty clear—the plates are getting bigger. But why?

To get this cultural backlash going, we need an enemy, something or somebody to fight against. A real, live conspiracy with evil corporate masterminds pulling the strings would be perfect.

So who's the villain? Did the manufacturers of America's tableware—Denby, Lenox, Fiesta, Royal Doulton, Wedgewood, and the rest—all gather in a room one day with all the grocery store bigwigs and decide they could make a buck selling us plates that are 30 percent larger than we actually need? Maybe. But unfortunately, I doubt it.

No, this was a little more gradual. A little more under our radar. Like when television screens went from 27 inches to 32, then from 40 inches to garage door size. Our plates just got a little bigger every decade or so, along with our middle-class appetite for "stuff." If there is a culprit behind the evil creation of Platezilla, it would have to be the restaurants. Restaurants have always known they can use bigger portions to make us feel like we're getting more value. For most restaurants, the food is the cheapest part of the experience. Believe it or not, it often costs more to wash the dishes than to pile food on them. Rent and labor and advertising (sorry) are expensive, too. But once you're sitting there, food is comparatively cheap. Pour on more. Those bigger portions demanded bigger plates. And those bigger plates looked so grand that pretty soon we also wanted them for our homes. You know, so we could have that "out to dinner" feeling every night. And because big had slowly and gradually become "normal"-looking. It wasn't your fault. It just happened.

We might want to take a pause here for a little disclaimer. Because although I say, "It wasn't your fault," I'm of the mind that anything that happens to us is our responsibility. Obviously, this goes against our society's "victim" mentality, but I'm still optimistic enough to believe we control our destiny. Not all of you will agree.

So the plates got bigger, and any eight-year-old could guess what happened next. We started putting more food on them. After all, the amount of food you would normally have served on a smaller plate suddenly looked pitiful and unfulfilling on a larger plate. And in our minds, if it doesn't look right, then it ain't right. So more room meant only one thing: more food. Mac and cheese. Meat loaf. Mashed potatoes and gravy. You name it. And, of course, more food meant more calories.

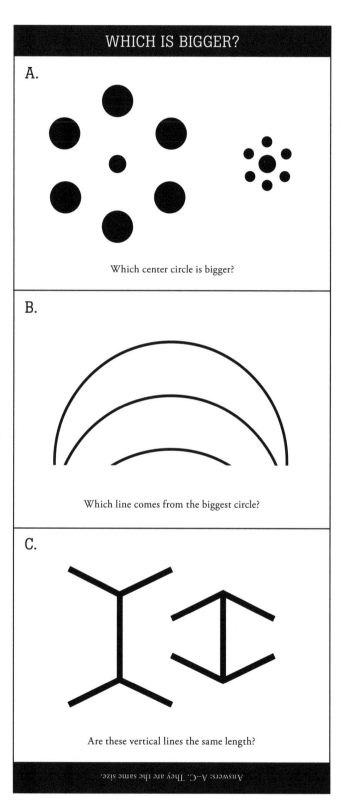

WHICH IS BIGGER?

A.

Which center circle is bigger?

B.

Which line comes from the biggest circle?

C.

Are these vertical lines the same length?

Answers: A–C: They are the same size.

SOME OF THESE TRICKS IN PERCEPTION ARE WELL DOCUMENTED. IT'S FUN STUFF AS A BRAIN TEASER. BUT IT KINDA SUCKS WHEN IT'S MAKING YOU FAT.

We're very visual animals, it turns out. In advertising photography if you want a small amount of food to look bigger, you put it on a smaller plate. Nobody would do it, but the inverse is also true. Put the same amount of food on a bigger plate, and it looks like less.

Some of these tricks in perception are well documented. It's fun stuff as a brain teaser. But it kinda sucks when it's making you fat.

And these plates full of food aren't just getting bigger. They're getting heavier with all the food it takes to make them look full. When you add it all up, we each ate 1,775 pounds of food in 2000—up from 1,497 pounds in 1970.

That's almost an additional 300 pounds of food per person—roughly the same weight as the average NFL offensive lineman. Since 1970, our plates have increased in size by about 20 percent, and our average caloric intake has increased by the same percentage. Maybe it's a coincidence, but I doubt it. As a friend of mine is fond of saying, "When I was a boy, I believed there were lots of coincidences. As a young man, I believed there were some coincidences. But now, I don't believe there is any such thing as coincidence."

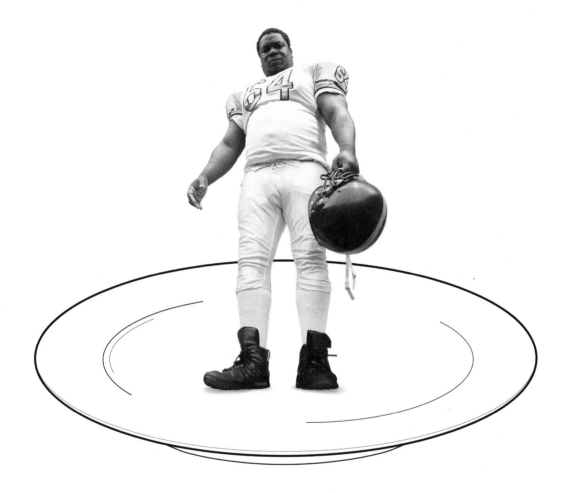

AMERICANS ATE 300 POUNDS MORE IN 2000 THAN THEY DID IN 1970. THAT'S THE WEIGHT OF AN AVERAGE NFL OFFENSIVE LINEMAN.

Source: LIFEhealth, *LIFE.info Magazine.* July 6, 2006.

The scales are tipping. Today, nearly 65 percent of the population is considered overweight, compared to 47 percent in 1970.

This caloric stuff is well documented. According to a recent report from the USDA, adult women are now eating 335 more calories per day than they did in 1971. Adult men have upped their daily intake by 168 calories. And contrary to popular opinion, it's not because of what we are eating, but because of how much we are eating.

With these kinds of numbers, many of us are starting to wonder why we ever thought bigger was better. The truth is, you probably never actually decided to think bigger is better. Nobody specifically gave you that choice to make. Our belief in bigness is so deeply rooted in American culture that it's just part of being a citizen of a country that stretches from one ocean to another. Manifest Destiny, baby. As a nation, we embraced bigness a long time ago. And those kinds of 200-year-old cultural myths die hard. Big cars. Big wheels. Big homes. Big belt buckles. Big hair. Bigness is about the quickest way we have of saying better. It's sort of shorthand for how we say success. Think about it. The single most affordable luxury for us all in this great land is to indulge in food. And the most basic form of indulgence is more.

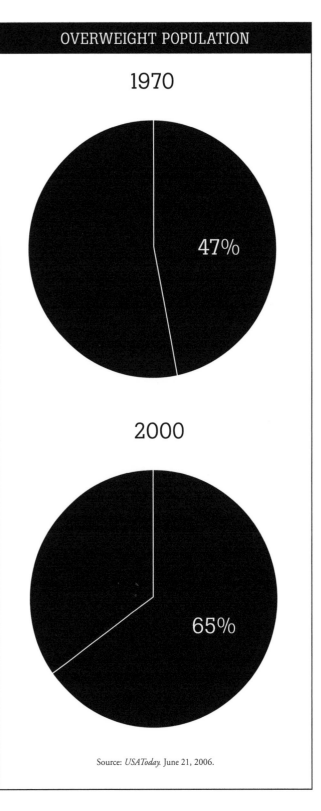

OVERWEIGHT POPULATION

1970

47%

2000

65%

Source: *USAToday.* June 21, 2006.

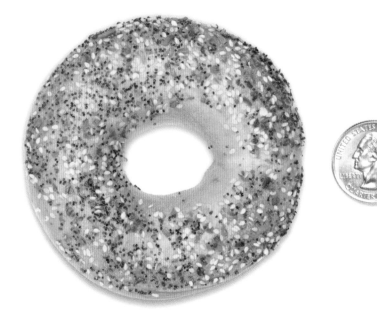

(BAGEL) 3-Inch Diameter, 140 Calories
20 Years Ago

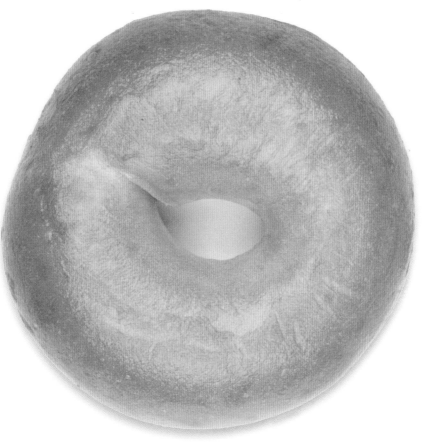

(BAGEL) 6-Inch Diameter, 350 Calories
Today

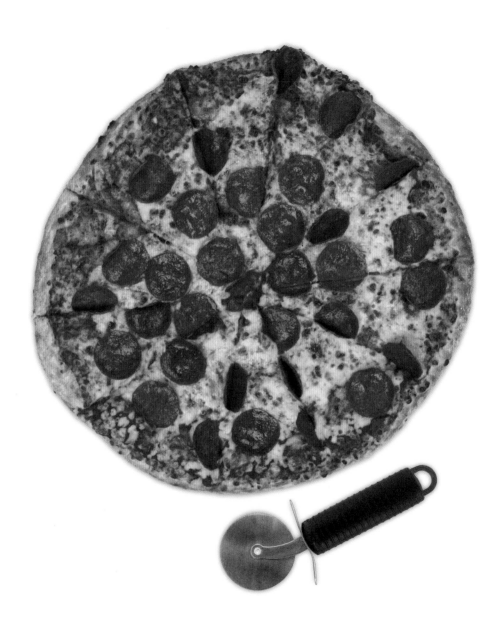

Pizza
20 Years Ago

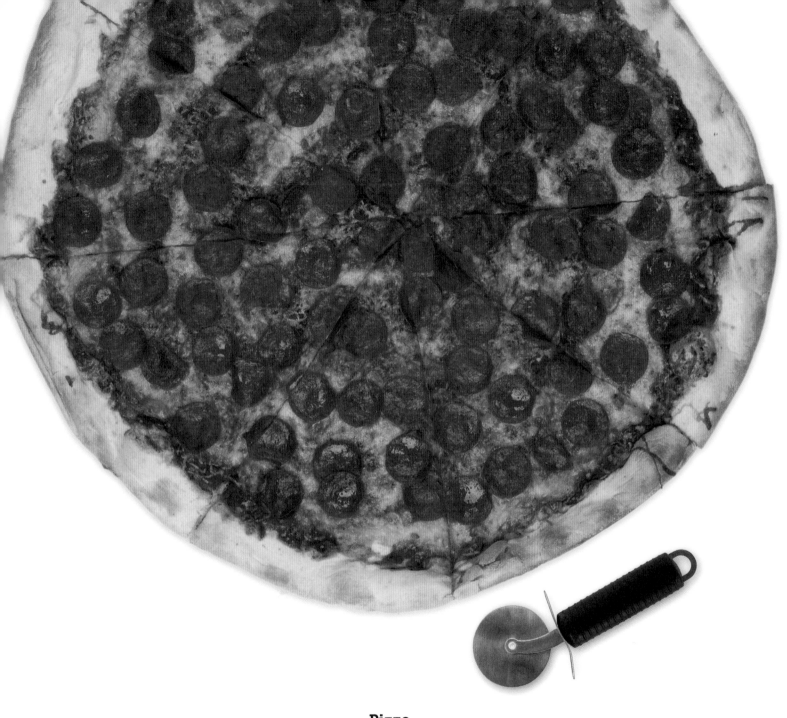

Pizza
Today

CHAPTER 2
WE'RE NOT STARVING IN AMERICA

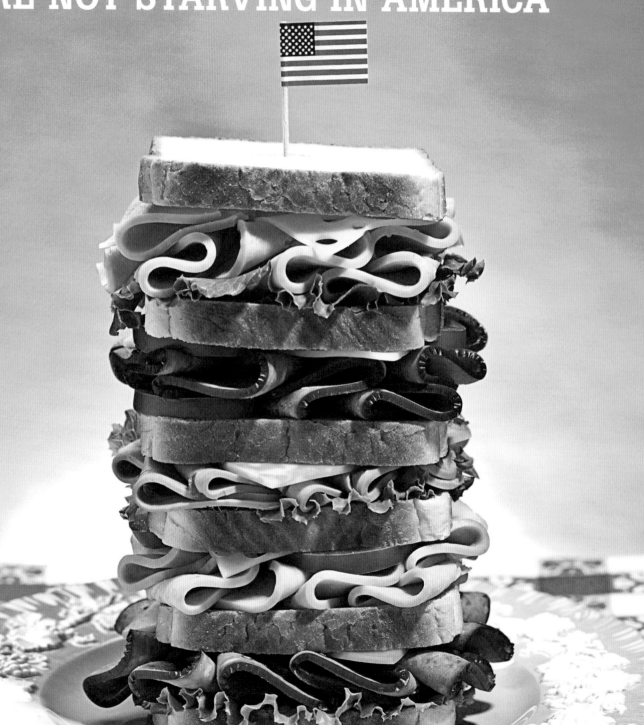

TO EAT A SMALL PORTION ACTUALLY MAKES YOU SUSPECT. YOU MIGHT BE A COMMUNIST. OR WORSE, FRENCH.

From the point of view of sociologists and anthropologists, the time that has passed since our society has gone from not having enough to eat to having the ability to overeat has been the blink of an eye. Being fat was a luxury of the rich at the turn of the century. It was fashionable. Even more recently, my grandparents didn't have enough to eat during the Great Depression. From a historical perspective, all this food is something new. And we obviously don't really know how to behave with this overabundance. We'll figure it out and get things back in balance. In a thousand years, I doubt many of us will be overweight. But what if you don't want to wait that long?

Our prosperity has not only meant more food on our tables at home, it has also meant that more and more of us can afford to eat out more and more often. And who doesn't love that? But as we all began to eat out more often, it set some dynamics in motion as restaurants competed for our business. It's doubtful that anybody in the restaurant business realized the effect their decisions were destined to have. They just knew that providing customers with huge portions was an affordable way to make them feel great about all they were getting for their money. It would be downright un-American to do it any other way. See how good it feels to think that way? That's the power of culture. In the beginning, those restaurants probably expected us to take half the food home in a doggie bag. They must have. But to everybody's surprise, we just went ahead and ate the whole thing. Without a second thought as to how much more we were eating. Why?

"We're getting so used to eating out and used to restaurants' portion sizes," says Lisa Drayer, a registered dietitian and the director of nutrition services with dietwatch.com, "we're getting a distorted view of what portion sizes are. We're not likely to make a distinction between restaurant sizes and real sizes when we go home."

And as big as the American plate is now, it's likely to get bigger. Getting more for your money is a powerful appeal, and every food marketer in America knows it.

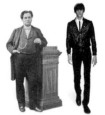

THE TIMES HAVE CHANGED: Being fat was a luxury of the rich at the turn of the century. It was fashionable then. It isn't today.

29

AND AS B
AMERICA
IS NOW, IT
TO GET

IG AS THE

N PLATE

S LIKELY

BIGGER.

CHAPTER 3
MEDIUM ISN'T A SIZE, IT'S AN IDEA

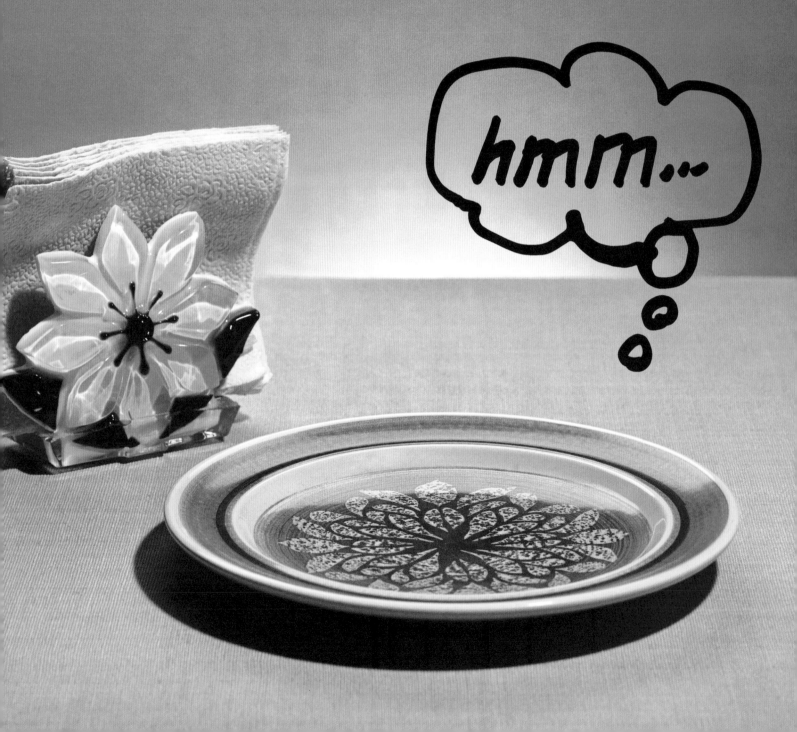

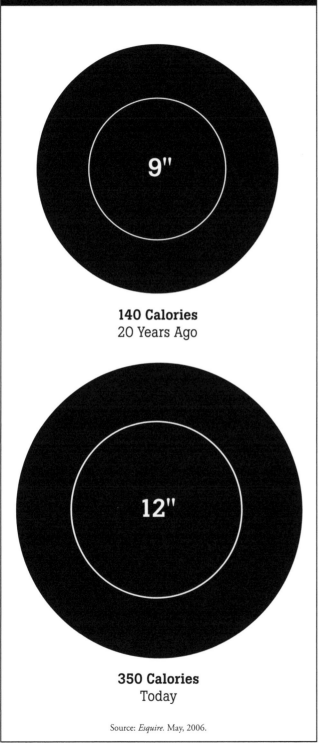

9"

140 Calories
20 Years Ago

12"

350 Calories
Today

Source: *Esquire.* May, 2006.

A DAY THAT SHALL LIVE IN INFAMY.

Some of you might be able to remember the day when movie theaters realized the power of oversized portions. I remember it vividly because it hit me right in the buttocks. Yes, the wallet. They raised prices as part of this scheme, and the price of my typical date night suddenly eclipsed the 20 bucks I had always budgeted (now you know I'm not only over 40, but also cheap). They got away with it, too. I've been waiting for this moment to call them on the carpet for 25 years. Payback is a bitch, movie theater folks. Deal with it.

Seemed like one moment you were buying a large soda at the theater snack counter and getting a 12-ounce beverage. Then suddenly (it might even have been when you ducked into the bathroom),

THE LARGE BECAME THE MEDIUM AND THE MEDIUM BECAME THE SMALL AND THE SMALL BECAME THE CHILD'S CUP.

there was a new "large" of 32 ounces. The large became the medium and the medium became the small and the small became the child's cup. And now, heck, they probably use that child's cup for samples or as a measuring spoon for the hot butter.

It may seem like we're all innocent victims of this elephantiasis of America, but we're the ones who nod "yes" when the cashier asks if we want the larger soda for only 35 cents more. Why? Because the system is designed to make us feel we've been ripped off if we buy the smaller size—and that we're really being quite moderate in choosing the medium—when, in fact, the medium is one or two sizes larger than what we used to consider medium. It's all about perception. Because the fact is, medium isn't a size. It's an idea. (You might want to take a moment here, because this is heavy.) And the size and shape of that idea have been changed to the point that we don't know what medium is anymore. You might think you do. I know how you tend to overestimate yourself, just like I do. But there is plenty of research that proves neither of us knows our medium from a hole in the ground.

My grandfather, who was a tough cuss from Oklahoma, was fond of telling me, "You don't know your ass from a hole in the ground, and I can prove it." Contrary to the tone of this anecdote, my grandfather and I loved each other as much as any grand pair that has come before or since. But he'd still get me. He would take a stick and he'd make a hole in the dirt and he'd say, "Now this is your ass. Got it?" Then he'd make another hole and say, "And this is a hole in the ground. Now which one is your ass?" I would of course pick the first hole and he would say, "I told you you didn't know your ass from a hole in the ground."

MEDIUM ISN'T A SIZE. IT'S AN IDEA.

I swear that I never got it while he was alive. He must have really worried about his dumb grandson because he never explained it to me, and I was in my 20s before it clicked. But I imagine it was his way of explaining to me not to believe something just because somebody is telling you it's true.

So just because somebody says to you that something is "medium-size" doesn't mean it's your idea of medium or mine or anyone else's. There has always

Brownlee writes, "Portion sizes have been creeping upward since 1972, when McDonald's introduced its large-size fries."

Of course, large is also a relative term. At 3.5 ounces, the 1972 "large" was smaller than a "medium" serving today. This is worth stating again. The 1972 "large" was smaller than the "medium" we buy today. And the crazy thing is that "large" looked large to everybody who ordered it and ate it. This is worth

MORE IS MORE: While it only costs pennies to increase the size of a portion, customers will pay at least a quarter more to buy it. And those quarters add up.

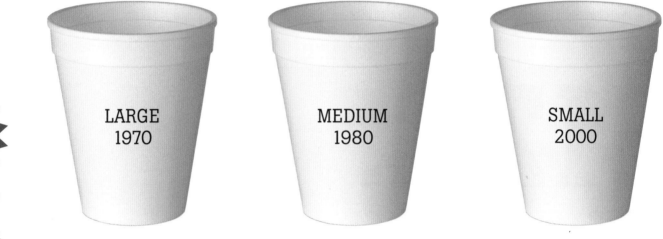

LARGE 1970   MEDIUM 1980   SMALL 2000

been this understanding that medium is the size that an average person seeking a moderate portion can safely order. This just isn't true anymore. In fact, the only thing you can be sure of about a medium is that it is the size in between the small and large.

If Americans really wanted to be smart about it, we'd throw away the entire notion of small, medium, and large and just go by actual size. Name a drink after the number of ounces.

In an article for *The Washington Post,* Shannon

restating, too. That 3.5-ounce portion appeared to be large when our 1972 brains saw it, but today we would laugh at somebody with the nerve to call that a large. And here's another thing that's true. If we took one of today's large-size fries back in time to 1972, they'd think we were sick to want that many fries in a single sitting.

Size is completely, utterly, and totally relative.

Now, before you start bashing McDonald's you should know that it actually increased its portions

THE DEAL IS SIMPLE: "WE'LL GIVE YOU A LOT MORE STUFF FOR JUST A LITTLE MORE MONEY."

reluctantly. The company's founder, Ray Kroc, didn't like the image of lowbrow, cheap food in huge portions. If people wanted more French fries, he would say, "They can buy two bags." Ray made a lot of sense, and we can only wish today he had won that argument back then. But price competition had become so fierce that the only way to keep profits up was to offer bigger and bigger portions. Burger King, Wendy's, and Taco Bell were all cutting their prices, selling more food, and making bigger profits while doing so. After all, it costs pennies to increase the size of a portion, but customers will pay at least a quarter more to buy it. And those quarters add up. By 1988, McDonald's had introduced a 32-ounce "super-size" soda and "super-size" fries. To put that into perspective, a classic bottle of Coke is 6.5 ounces. So, we can now order one cup that contains five 1970 Coca-Cola portions.

If you saw somebody with a burger and five bottles of Coke you might think it a bit odd, even today. But the big cup makes it "normal."

In the corporate world, this phenomenon has a name—value marketing. The deal is simple: "We'll give you a lot more stuff for just a little more money." That would be great if we were all sumo wrestlers and actually needed those huge portions. The fact is, we don't need the extra calories. Our bodies can't burn them over the course of the day, and so we store the excess as fat. Of course, we're the ones responsible for what we put in our bodies. This isn't a blame game. But it is obvious that our psychological makeup means we'll fall for this size game again and again and again and again and again. As my son would say, "Again infinity." We're just not equipped to perceive quantities without comparison. A medium will always be defined by the relative size of a large and a small and not by any truly rational measurement. Over the millions of years since we first stood upright, our brains have developed us as hunter/gatherers. Not as hunter/gatherer/measurers.

And it's not just me saying this. According to Melanie Polk, the director of nutrition education at the American Institute for Cancer Research, "Value marketing has confused Americans about what a 'normal' and appropriate portion of food should look like."

NORMAL
–adjective
1. conforming to the standard or the common type; usual; not abnormal; regular; natural.

YOU DON
YOUR M
FROM A
THE G

T KNOW
EDIUM
HOLE IN
ROUND.

CHAPTER 4
HEY, LOOK—A MAYONNAISE JAR BIGGER THAN YOUR HEAD

IN A CULTURE OF BIGNESS, IT IS HARD TO EMBRACE SMALL. HELL, IT'S HARD TO FIND SMALL.

There are plenty of other portion distortion culprits besides the drive-thru window. Wholesale clubs, like Costco and Sam's Club, confuse us. We think, no, of course we won't eat that huge industrial-size jar of Cheez Whiz in one sitting. But the funny thing is, the larger size makes us lose our perspective and ultimately our inhibitions. We're using more from these larger containers, and we can't help it and don't even know it. We can't know it. We aren't designed to know it. We are creating a world around ourselves that conspires to take advantage of the limitations in our perceptual makeup.

In an award-winning research study that was quoted in *The Wall Street Journal* and *Harvard Business Review*, University of Illinois psychologist Brian Wansink showed that a larger package size can accelerate the use of a product by anywhere from 7 to 43 percent. Study participants who were told to prepare a dinner for two pulled out 29 percent more spaghetti noodles when using a larger box and poured 23 percent more oil to fry chicken when using a larger bottle. (And it's not just food. Participants used 11 percent more laundry detergent from a large box compared to a small one. In fact, five studies with 691 adults across 47 product categories showed that people virtually always use more of a product if it's in a larger package rather than a small one.) Wansink says, "Buying foods in bulk makes us eat more. We seem to think that because we can get something in five-gallon tubs, it must be OK to eat larger quantities. Also, the need to conserve food is gone because we see that we've got plenty to spare."

But all of this isn't really about what we think because pretty much all of this is happening outside of any kind of analytic thought. It is instinct and impulse, and we're out of control.

In a culture of bigness, it is hard to embrace small. Hell, it's hard to find small.

"Today," says Lisa Young, a nutritionist at New York University, "super-sizing has pervaded every segment of the food industry. Portion sizes over the years have ballooned, and it's no coincidence that people are gaining weight." For her PhD, Young documented the changes in portion sizes for dozens of foods over the past several decades. M&M/Mars, for example, has increased the size of candy bars, such as Milky Way and Snickers, four times since 1970. Starbucks introduced the twenty-ounce "venti" size in 1999 and discontinued its "short" eight-ounce cup. When 22-ounce Heinekens were introduced, Young

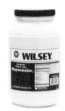

ABOVE:
I love mayonnaise sandwiches. This is probably enough for several lifetimes.

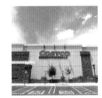

ABOVE:
Popping up everywhere from suburbia to the city are wholesale clubs, like Sam's Club and Costco. These stores pride themselves on *"The bigger, the better."*

41

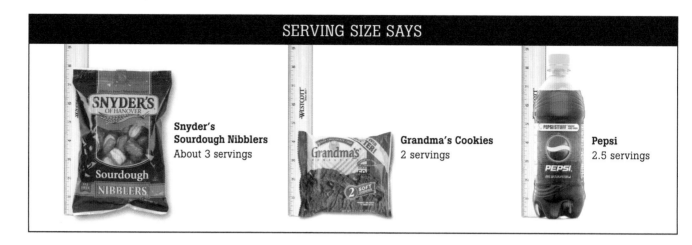

Snyder's Sourdough Nibblers
About 3 servings

Grandma's Cookies
2 servings

Pepsi
2.5 servings

reported, the company sold 24 million of them the first year and attributed the sales to the "big-bottle gimmick." Even Lean Cuisine and Weight Watchers now advertise "hearty portions" of their diet meals.

But it's not just food that's been getting bigger. It's America. The average square footage of new homes has been steadily increasing for 40 years. There are master bathrooms now bigger than the living rooms most of us grew up in. The average TV screen size increased from 14 inches to 17, and then to 21 inches by the 1970s. In the 80s and 90s, the main family TV set went from 27 inches to 40 inches. And now you can buy a TV with a 70-inch screen. That is, if you can fit it through your front door. How ridiculous does an eight-ounce Coke bottle look in your hand as you sit in front of a 70-inch screen in your chair-and-a-half?

Pick up an eight-ounce Coke sometime if you can find one. It looks stupidly small. You'll laugh. And when you stop laughing, you'll realize that you have been convinced by comparison that a "normal"-size portion is laughably small. Not good.

For most beverages and ready-to-eat foods, market-ers are required to put nutritional and dietary information on the package. But one particularly tricky part of the whole portion distortion game is trying to figure out how many portions are in a package or a bottle. Older people tend to do better at this than younger people because they can still remember when there were "normal"-size candy bars, single-serving bags of peanuts, and eight-ounce Cokes. I barely remember those days, and if you're younger than me, I'm betting you can't remember them at all.

In fact, in one study published in the *Journal of the American Board of Family Medicine,* only 37 percent of those tested could determine the number of servings in snack food packages. Take the test on the next page and let's see how you do.

It's simple. Big packages make you think it's OK to eat more. Three servings in one package make you think three servings are what you're supposed to be eating.

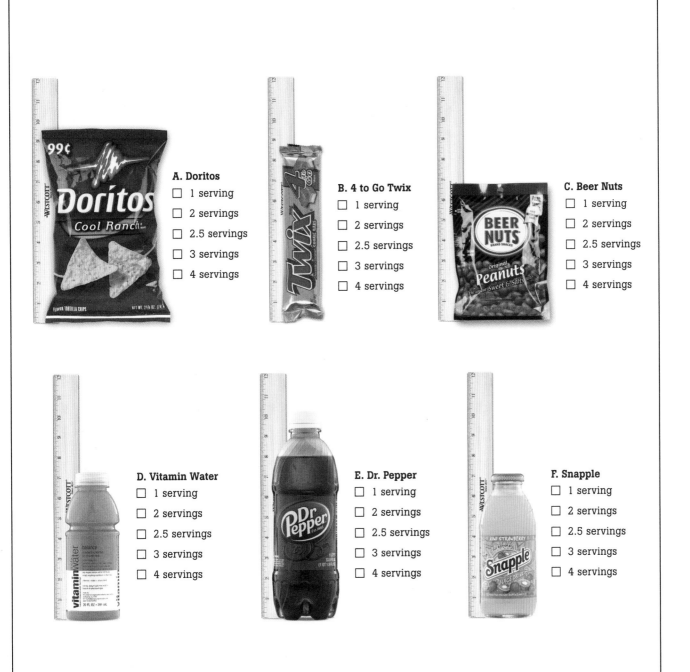

A. Doritos
- ☐ 1 serving
- ☐ 2 servings
- ☐ 2.5 servings
- ☐ 3 servings
- ☐ 4 servings

B. 4 to Go Twix
- ☐ 1 serving
- ☐ 2 servings
- ☐ 2.5 servings
- ☐ 3 servings
- ☐ 4 servings

C. Beer Nuts
- ☐ 1 serving
- ☐ 2 servings
- ☐ 2.5 servings
- ☐ 3 servings
- ☐ 4 servings

D. Vitamin Water
- ☐ 1 serving
- ☐ 2 servings
- ☐ 2.5 servings
- ☐ 3 servings
- ☐ 4 servings

E. Dr. Pepper
- ☐ 1 serving
- ☐ 2 servings
- ☐ 2.5 servings
- ☐ 3 servings
- ☐ 4 servings

F. Snapple
- ☐ 1 serving
- ☐ 2 servings
- ☐ 2.5 servings
- ☐ 3 servings
- ☐ 4 servings

Answers: A. 3 servings, B. 4 servings, C. 3 servings, D. 2.5 servings, E. 4 servings, F. 2 servings.

CHAPTER 5
SURPRISE, YOUR EYES REALLY ARE BIGGER THAN YOUR STOMACH

IT TAKES BETWEEN TEN AND TWENTY MINUTES FOR THE STOMACH TO TELL THE BRAIN IT'S FULL. HOW MUCH EXTRA FOOD CAN YOU EAT IN TEN TO TWENTY MINUTES?

I've already talked about some of the findings of Brian Wansink, the consumer psychology expert from the University of Illinois. He's the one who originally coined the phrase "portion distortion" to describe how our eyes often fool our stomach. It explains why we roll our eyes when we're served what looks like a little bit of food on a great big plate in a chic restaurant. And why, conversely, we may feel perfectly satisfied when eating the same portion off a smaller plate. The reality is that we're just not equipped as humans to make rational judgments about the portions we eat. Wansink didn't invent portion distortion; he just proved it's for real.

In various experiments he demonstrated that—without visual cues to remind us when we've eaten enough—the more we're served, the more we'll eat. In one experiment, Wansink's team studied a number of people at (What else?) a Super Bowl party. Researchers served platters of chicken wings, then cleared the plates off some tables but left plates with chicken bones sitting out on others. When they tallied how much each group consumed, they found that when they continually cleared the tables—removing the evidence of how much had already been eaten—the groups ate 24 percent more.

In a separate experiment with trick soup bowls (Wouldn't you love to have trick soup bowls?), participants who ate out of bowls that were automatically refilled by an unseen tube under the table ate 40 to 70 percent more soup. 70 percent. That means some people ate nearly twice as much soup before their stomachs told them they'd had enough. The practical problem here is that with the size of the average soup bowl today, we actually do have trick soup bowls. They hold more than a sensible portion, and we can't resist filling them up so that they look full.

It takes between 10 and 20 minutes for the stomach to tell the brain it's full. How much extra food can you eat in 10 to 20 minutes?

These experiments seem to show that our feelings of hunger could be more mental than physical. People who had a visual cue that they'd had enough to eat ate less than those who did not, which means their hunger was turned off by their perceptions before it was triggered to be turned off by a full stomach. The implication is that if we wait for our stomachs to tell us we're full, we will be eating too much. This is huge news about why we're getting huge.

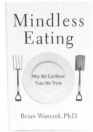

ABOVE:
Brian Wansink's book *Mindless Eating* explores our eating habits.

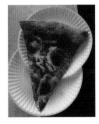

ABOVE:
When you regain some portion of sanity you start to see the insanity around you. I had to laugh recently when I got a piece of pizza so big it was served on two plates. Maybe soon we can all sit on two chairs while we eat.

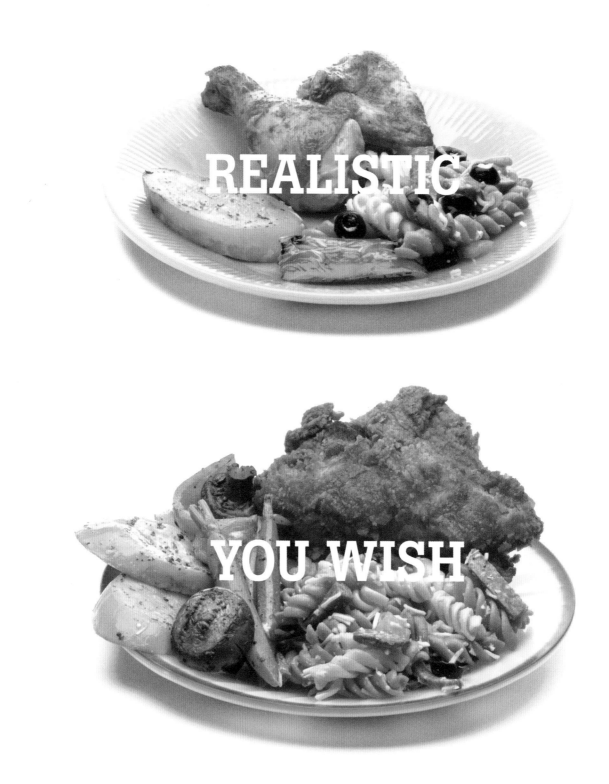

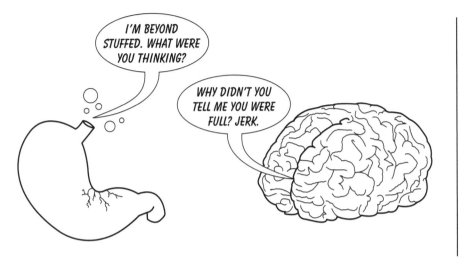

It takes between 10 and 20 minutes for the stomach to tell the brain it's full.

If we wait for our stomach to tell us we're full, we will be eating too much.

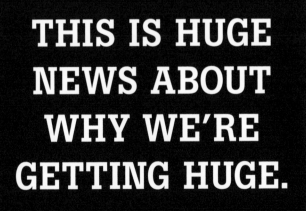

THIS IS HUGE NEWS ABOUT WHY WE'RE GETTING HUGE.

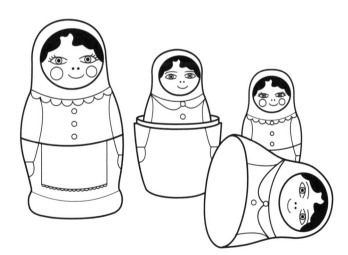

CHAPTER 6
SIZE MATTERS

Seeing evidence of how much we have eaten isn't the only cue our brain uses when it tells us how much to eat. Other studies by our old pal Wansink showed that the size and shape of plates and glasses can alter our perceptions of the amounts they hold.

When asked to pour the same amount of liquid into a tall, skinny glass and a short, wide glass, bartenders poured more into the short glass, believing that the two amounts looked equal. The fact is our eyes can, and do, fool us. They think it's fun.

Studies that began way back in the 30s have shown that when we view objects of exactly the same size, triangles are perceived to be larger than squares, squares larger than circles, and elongated objects larger than less elongated objects. Like I said before, we're very visual animals but our eyes often fool us. Is it any wonder we have trouble figuring out what size portion is bigger or smaller?

Also, according to Wansink, "External cues, such as packaging and container size, can powerfully and unknowingly increase how much food a person consumes." I know we keep coming back to movie theaters, but it's not just because they kept me broke when I was a kid. Wansink actually conducted another experiment there. His team randomly gave moviegoers either a medium-size popcorn or a large-size popcorn for free. And they weren't for sharing—each person in the party got one. After the movie, the containers were collected and weighed to determine how much popcorn had been eaten. The results? People ate an average of 53 percent more popcorn from a large container than from a medium container. Why am I not surprised?

USDA statistics show that America's total daily caloric intake has risen from 1,854 calories to 2,002 calories in the past 20 years. The solution is simple. Eat less. But with portion distortion wreaking havoc on our psyche, it's easier said than done. You might say that the system is actually designed to make us fail.

By now you might be thinking, since manipulating perception, distorting reality, and downright visual trickery play such an important role in how much we eat, maybe an advertising guy is exactly who should be writing a diet book.

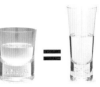

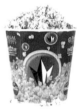

ABOVE:
Size and shape of the container can influence how much we eat or drink.

BELOW:
The larger the serving size, the more people will eat.

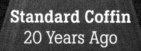

Standard Coffin
20 Years Ago

"SUPER-SIZE" THAT. THE NEW MEDIUM IN CASKETS IS 20% LARGER THAN THE OLD STANDARD SIZE.

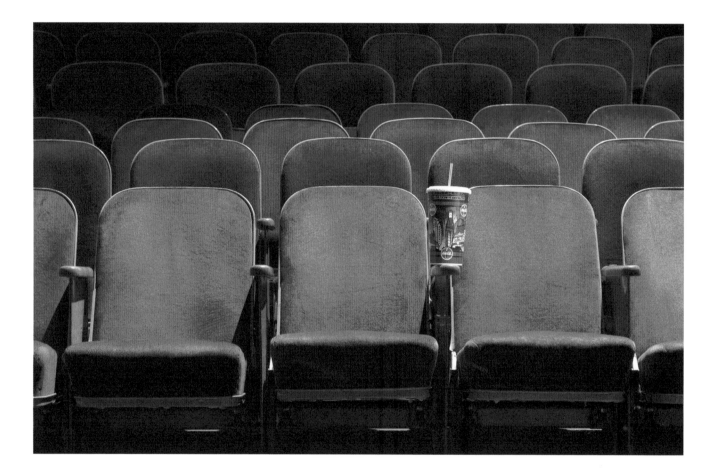

Movie Theater
20 Years Ago

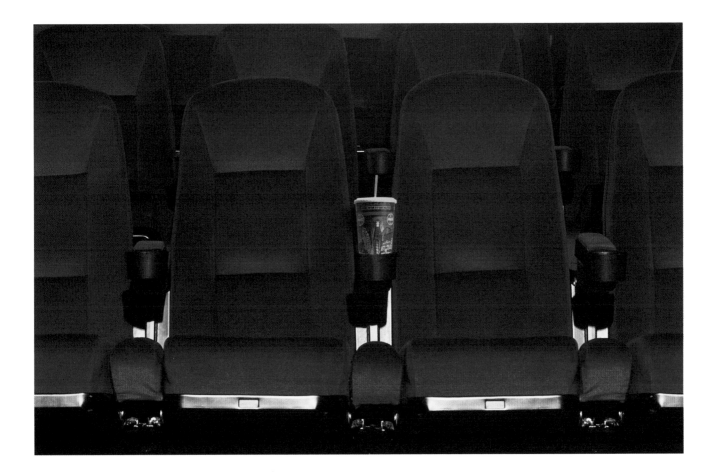

Movie Theater
Today

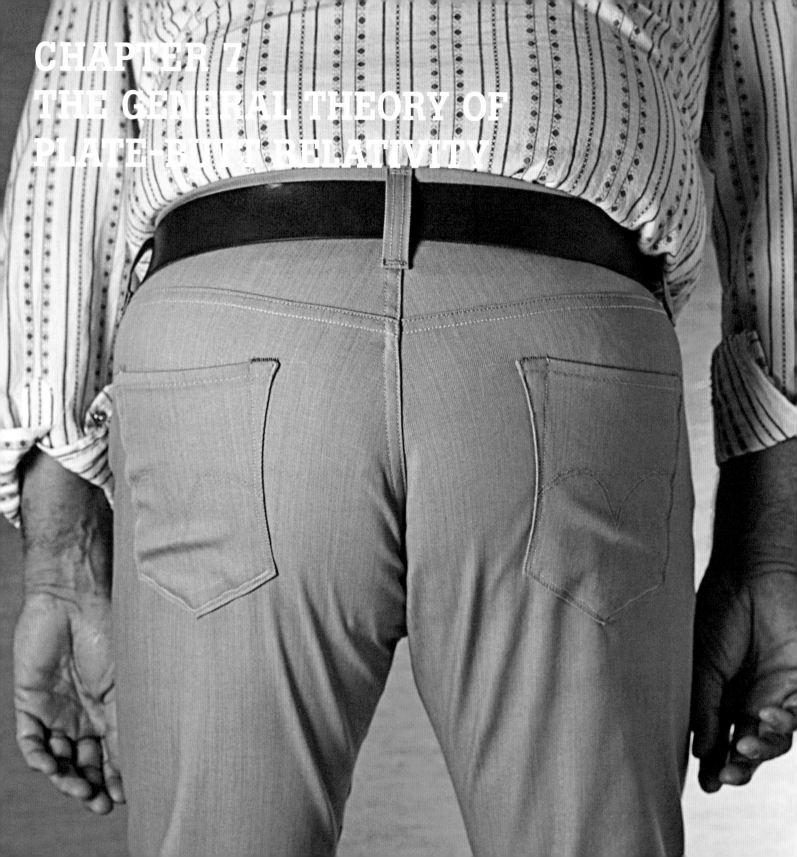

CHAPTER 7
THE GENERAL THEORY OF
PLATE-BUTT RELATIVITY

So where do all this extra food and all those extra calories end up? Well, here's a hint. Airplane seats have gradually become too small for airplane passengers.

Up until recently, most airline seats were designed based on a 1950 Harvard study of train passengers that had said the average adult required 18 inches per seat. So, most airliner seats, at least in coach, were always between 17 and 18 inches wide. And for decades, that was just fine. Well, next time you're wedged in a middle seat, tell me how fine it is. The BBC News World Edition, July 5, 2002, estimates that fully one-third of Americans cannot comfortably fit in the average airline seat. And about one person in 12 can't fit, period.

When Boeing was designing the new Boeing 777 in the late 80s, one of its key parameters was to make the plane wide enough so that the seats could be at least 18.5 inches across. At a minimum.

Many sports stadiums are increasing the width of their seats as well, along with auditoriums and concert halls. In the 2006 model, Honda widened its seats in the Civic by almost an inch "to accommodate the growing needs of our customers," according to a

ONE-THIRD OF AMERICANS CANNOT COMFORTABLY FIT IN THE AVERAGE AIRLINE SEAT. AND ABOUT ONE PERSON IN TWELVE CAN'T FIT, PERIOD.

company spokesperson. And I love this next one: In a classic piece of irony, the big movie theater chains have had to put in new seats—sometimes up to 24 inches across—so that the people who've been drinking their giant sodas and eating those tubs of popcorn for all these years can fit comfortably. I hope it has cost a ton.

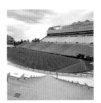

ABOVE:
The ripple effect of something like this is astounding. Start with a bigger plate and pretty soon your stadium seats are bigger, making entire stadiums bigger, and forcing Boeing to make a bigger plane to fly our butts from venue to venue.

From 1950 to today:
Three-inch bigger plates, 1.5-inch bigger butts.

(For every inch our plates have grown, our butts have
grown half an inch. Luckily, it should work
the same way on the way down.)

PLATE-BUTT RELATIVITY

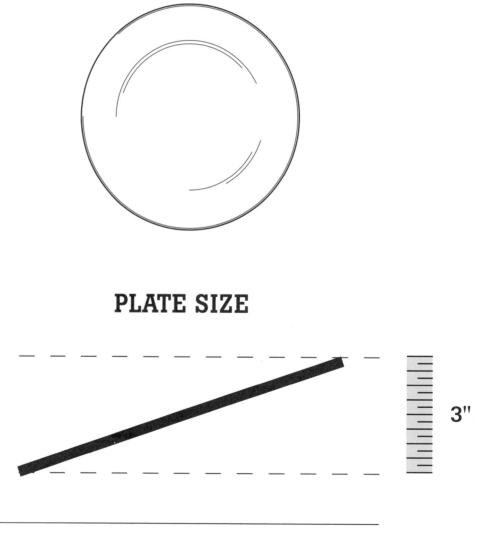

PLATE SIZE

1950   TODAY

3"

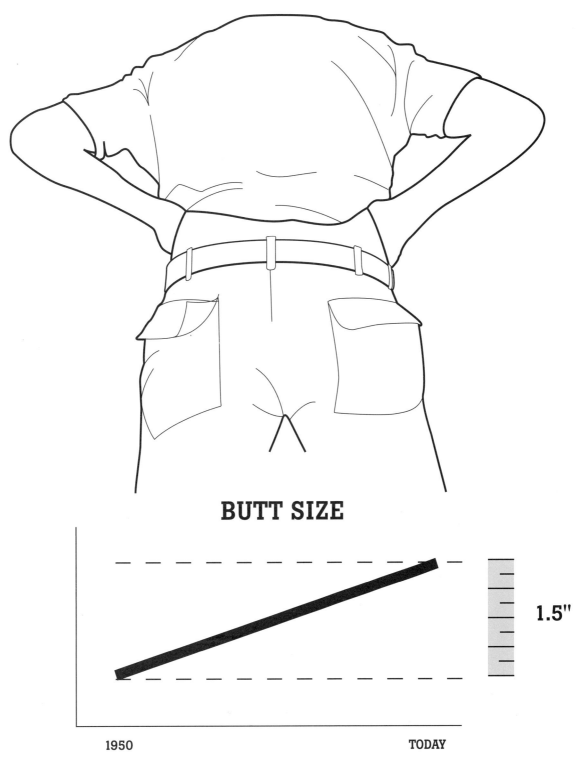

BUTT SIZE

1950   TODAY

1.5"

CHAPTER 8
IT'S A CONSPIRACY

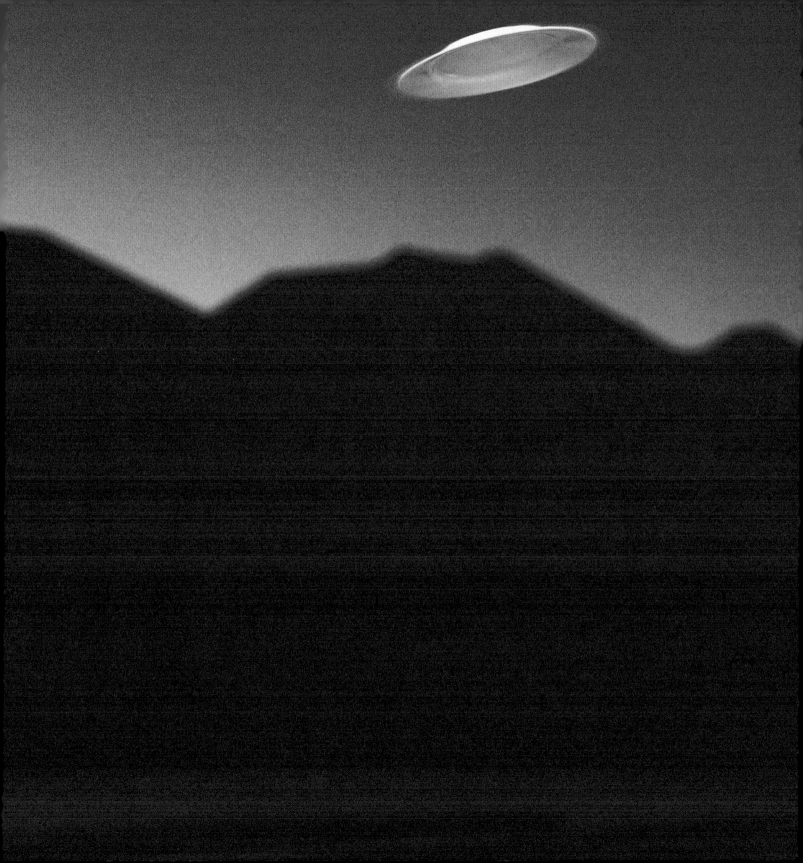

ALL OF US WHO DRINK THE NEW MEDIUM SODA NEED A NEW MEDIUM SHIRT TO GO WITH IT.

Obviously, our plates are getting bigger, our food is getting bigger, and we're getting bigger. All the facts prove it. Still, it's hard to admit and hard to accept. What we'd like to do is ignore the whole thing. Pretend it's not true. And today, thanks to the magic of marketing (Wasn't that a book title in the 50s?), that's just what we can do.

See, the apparel marketers are just as smart, and understand how to manipulate perception just as well as the food marketers—maybe more so. They know their customers buy clothes that make them feel good about themselves, express their personalities, give them a sense of style, and stroke their egos. But what they know more than anything else is that customers don't buy clothes that make them feel fat. That's Rule One.

All of us who drink the new medium soda need a new medium shirt to go with it.

Over the past 10 years, the average dress size has gone from a size eight to a size ten. But that's not the bad news. The bad news is that a size eight today is a hell of a lot bigger than a size eight used to be. It's portion distortion wearing a new spring outfit, and it's so common that it even has a name—vanity sizing. Kate Jackson of *The Boston Globe* reports that, on average, a dress size that would have been an eight in the 50s was a four in the 70s and is, today, a zero. It's the old put-four-Cokes-in-a-cup-but-call-it-a-medium trick, and it works like a dream. "Hey, it's not too much; it's a medium." "Hey, I'm not overweight; I'm a size six."

Guys are in a slightly better situation because of the Civil War. Back then, when the government had to make uniforms for a couple of million soldiers, it established sizing guidelines—based on real measurements in real inches—that are, for the most part, still in use for men's clothing today. Unless you're playing the small, medium, large, extra-large game. In college, I used to wear an extra-large. It was a little big, but comfortable. In reality, I was probably a large. Today, I'm finding I need to go with a medium, and with some brands, I'm even rocking a small. I'm five feet, ten inches and 170 pounds. Not a large man, but a small? I wish.

Vanity sizing has become so rampant, and garments that are now called a size zero (or even double-zero) have become so large, that women who really would have been a size zero a few years back now report difficulty in finding clothes that fit. There's even been talk in the industry about going to negative sizes. Now that is hilarious. Hilarious in an "if we didn't laugh, we would cry" kind of way.

What vanity sizing really does is make sizes, well, bullshit. Ben Whitford of Columbia News Service found that a 30-inch waist skirt was a size six at Anne Klein, a size four at Nine West, and a size two at French Connection. Maybe that's the real reason the French don't have to diet.

Obviously, that little size number has a huge psychological effect no matter who you are. Rumors are that one very A-list celeb has the size cut out of every garment she buys and has a size four tag sewn in.

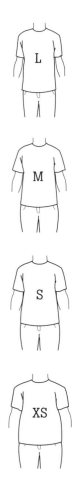

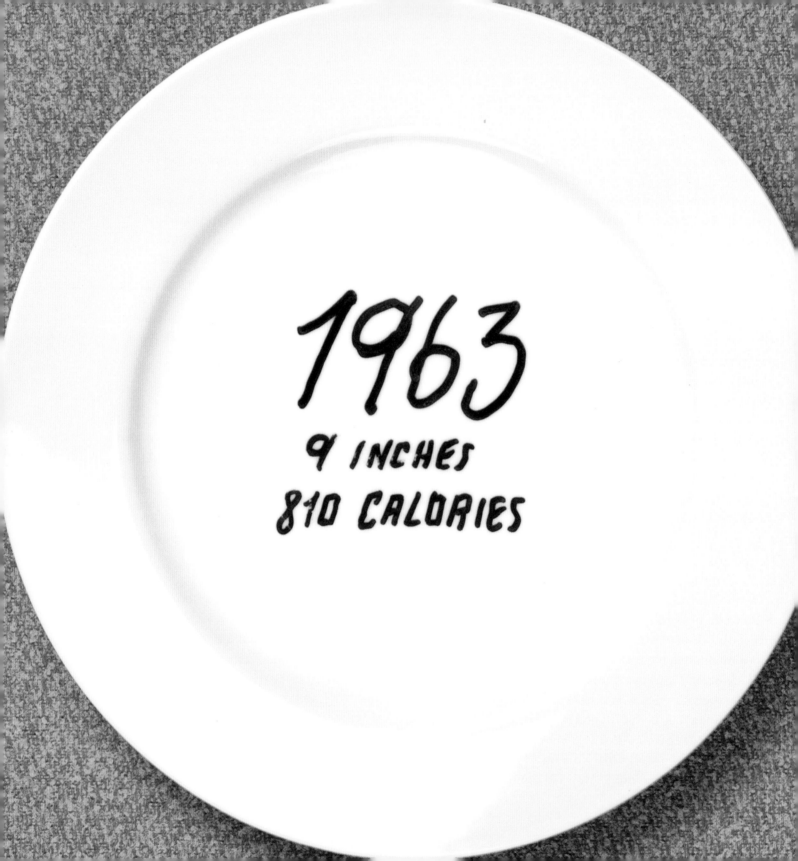

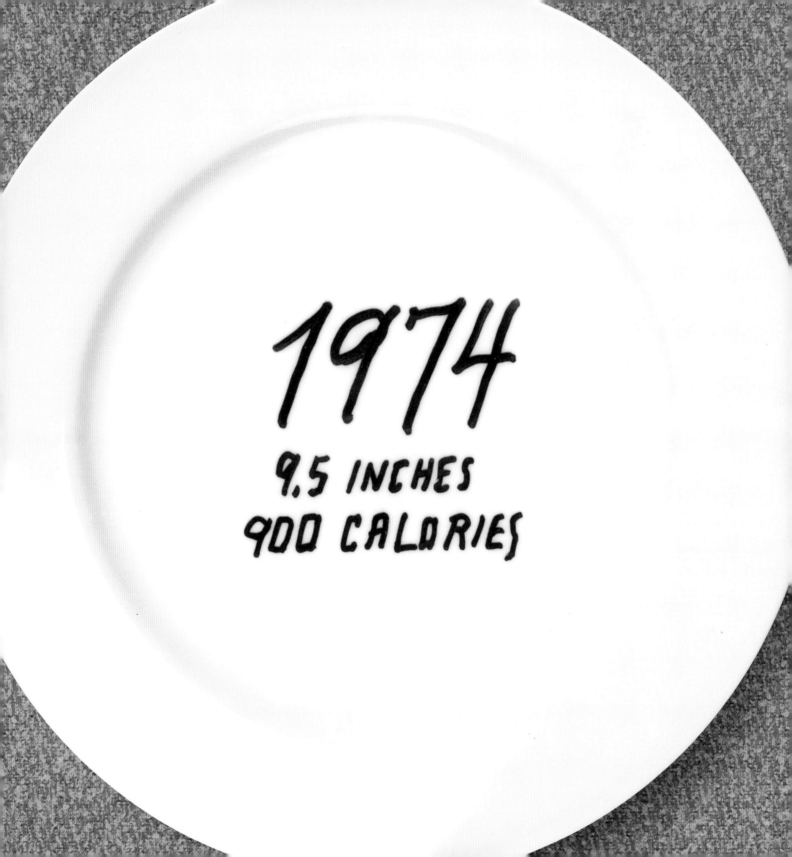

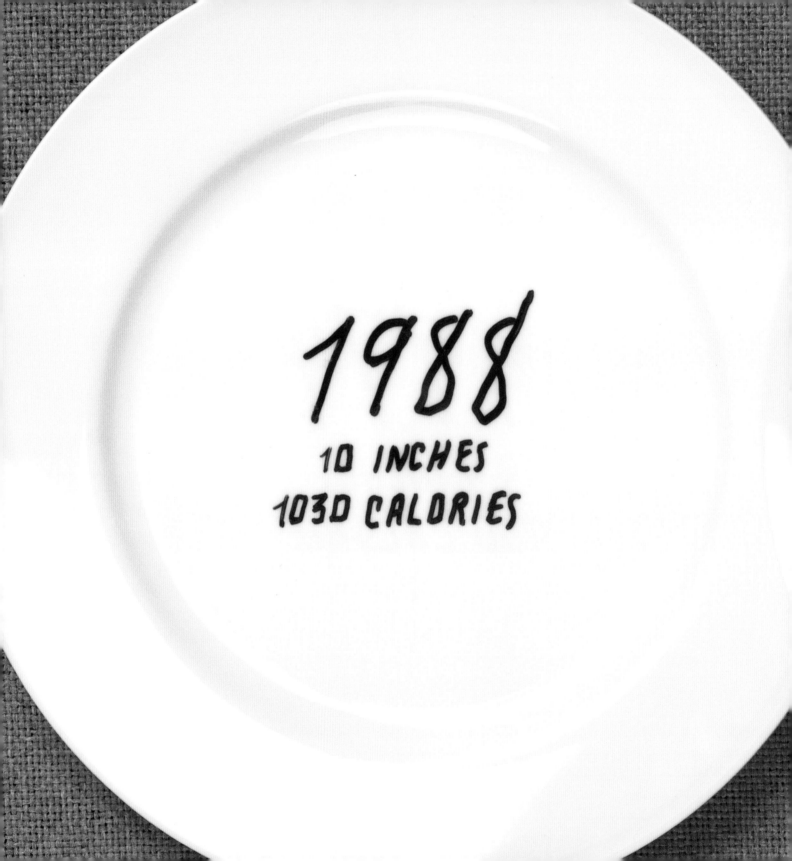

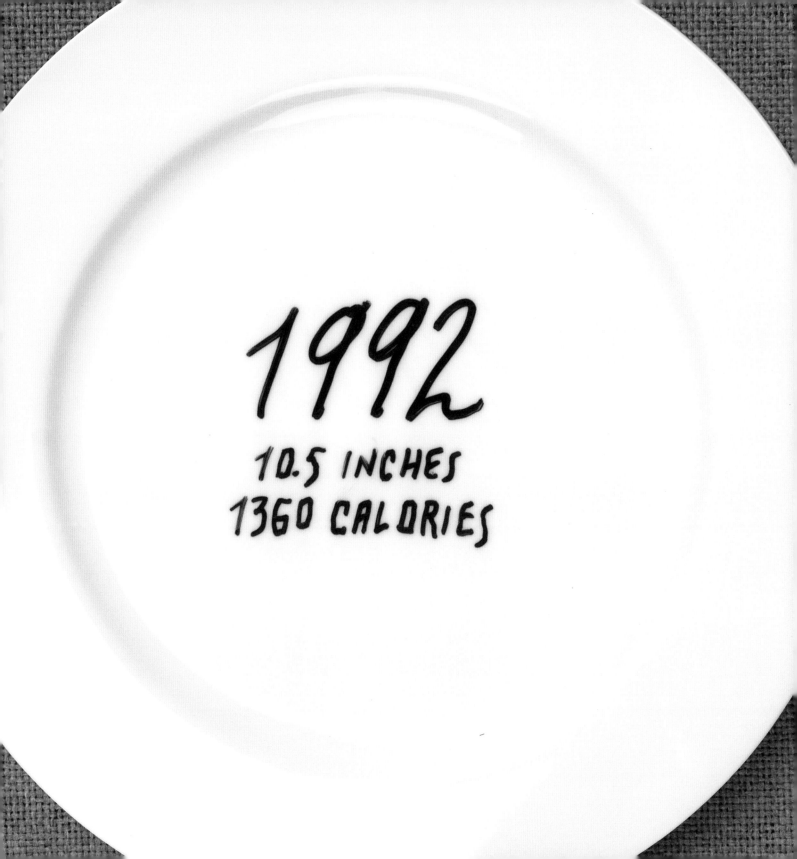

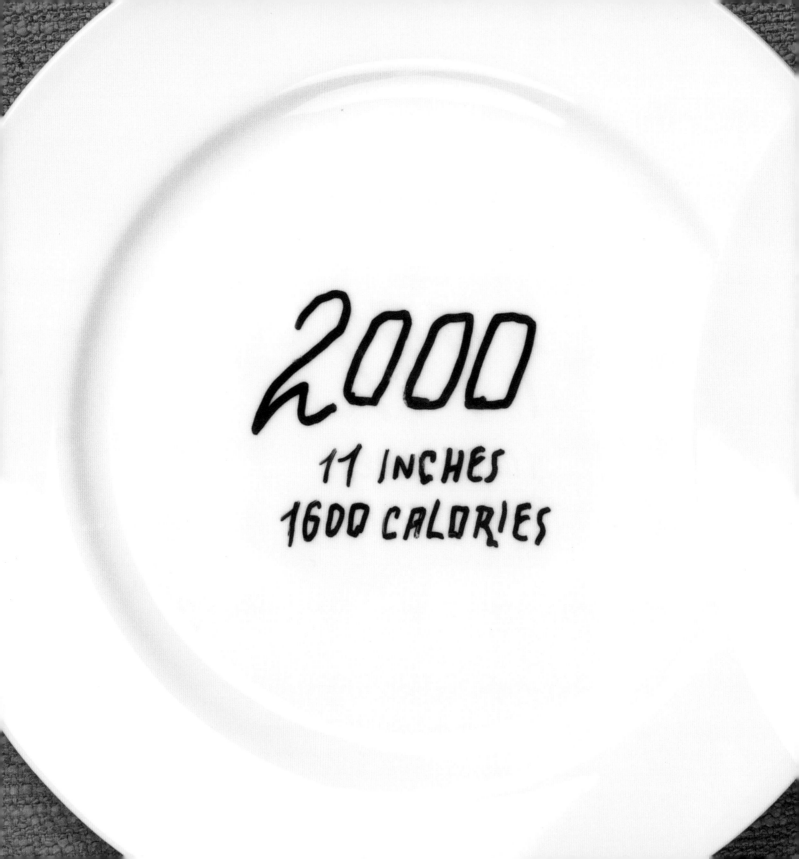

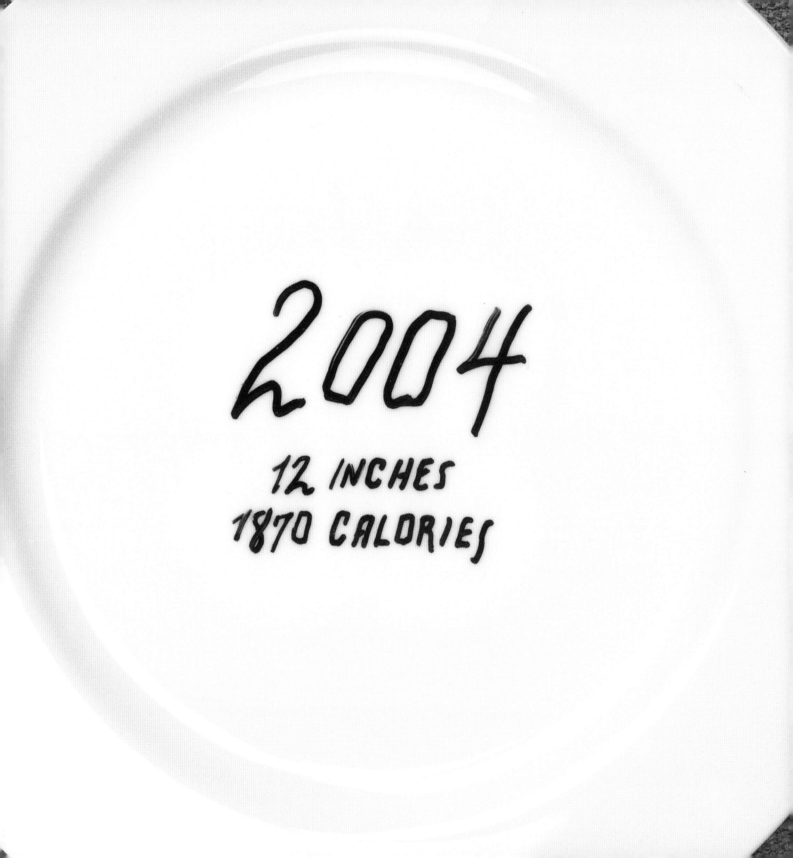

2004

12 INCHES
1870 CALORIES

CHAPTER 9
AS USUAL, YOU CAN BLAME EITHER YOUR PARENTS OR THE GOVERNMENT

By now, at least some of you are thinking, "This is nuts. Who cares what size the plate is? You don't have to eat it all."

Well, it turns out that for most people—for a whole bunch of reasons—not eating it all is a very hard thing to do. Partly because eating is a pretty fundamental impulse—if you don't, you die. But a lot of studies also show that the reluctance to leave leftovers on the plate is something that is programmed into us as we grow up. In fact, research conducted by Barbara Rolls, a physiologist at Penn State University, found that babies and toddlers aren't affected by portion size at all. "It doesn't matter how much you try to serve them; they stop eating when they're full."

In her experiment, Rolls tested three- to five-year-old kids to see which of the children would be influenced by the portions served to them. The results? The younger children stopped eating when they were full, no matter how much food was left on their plates. But the older children responded like adults. The bigger the portion, the more they ate.

(Here's another non-diet book observation. Babies are fat. And they're supposed to be fat. They have those cute insie knuckles. Attention: This book is not for babies. If you're a baby and you've somehow learned to read already, please close this book immediately.)

In a chat on WebMD, Rolls explains, "Young children respond to their physical hunger, while older kids, like adults, react to external cues." She believes that many parents condition their children to eat more with the "clean plate club" mentality and guilt trips like, "Think of the starving kids in China." I still think of that every time I have moo goo gai pan.

Anyway, we grow up thinking it's wasteful to leave anything on our plates. And, if your family is like mine, you learn to like the praise when you finish every last bite. It's amazing how powerful this is. Here I am, writing this book, and I still find myself doling out the "nice job" when the plate is cleaned. Lucky for my kids, they're eating off nine-inch plates.

In the end, most of us view finishing our plate as an accomplishment. Finishing is the goal.

But your parents don't get the whole rap for this.

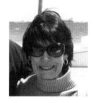

ABOVE:
My mom,
Dixie Bogusky.

WHO ELSE IS TO BLAME? THE GOVERNMENT. NATURALLY.

Who else is to blame? The government. Naturally.

In August of 1917, Congress passed the Food and Fuel Control Act. The main purpose of the act was to help the country avoid food shortages during World War I and to limit food imports so that we'd have more money for tanks. President Wilson put future president Herbert Hoover (who stepped into the ring at a hefty 210 pounds, and I'm not making that up) in charge of the U.S. Food Administration.

Hoover had a plan. According to author Kelly Burgess, "The idea was to conserve food by self-rationing scarce foods, such as flour and sugar, and encouraging people to focus on eating what they put on their plates so that nothing went to waste. In order to get the message out, he relied heavily on America's sense of volunteerism and patriotism." He distributed pledge cards to the public, requesting that every man, woman, and child make a solemn oath to save as much food as possible. Local newspapers kept running tallies of the households that had signed on, so the social pressure to join up and clean your plate was enormous. Schoolchildren signed pledges that had a little easy-to-remember rhyme:

"At the table, I'll not leave a scrap of food upon my plate. And I'll not eat between meals, but for suppertime I'll wait."

Funny how today, if a nutritionist crafted a message to kids, it would more than likely be the opposite of this one.

The Food Administration even created its own ad campaign, which positioned the "clean plate" as part of the American way.

Even after war rationing was over, the portrayal of a clean plate as the American ideal persisted. A clean plate was a good plate. A clean plate meant you were doing right by your country. The whole idea was reinforced during the Second World War and the rebuilding that followed. Just after the war, President Truman called upon the country to eat less as a way to save food for "thousands of starving Europeans."

A campaign was launched to create "clean plate clubs" in elementary schools all across America. That was 60 years ago, and you probably never saw the ads yourself. But if you've ever heard the expression "clean plate," you can chalk another one up to the incredibly long-lasting power of advertising.

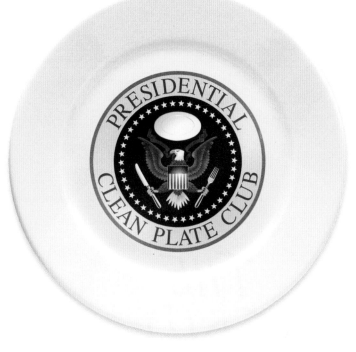

"One poll showed that seven out of ten Americans will still clean their plate regardless of how much is on it," says Julie Matthews, a certified nutrition consultant and the author of *Healthful Living*. "So what was originally introduced as an incentive for Americans to conserve food and eat less has become an unhealthy habit."

In defense of the "clean plate clubs," I should also note that we were being asked to clean an 8.5- or 9-inch plate. Even the government wouldn't suggest we be cleaning off the huge-ass plates of today. "The notion of 'cleaning your plate' was originally tied to another equally important idea: Put only what you need on your plate in the first place," says Melanie Polk, director of nutrition at the American Institute for Cancer Research.

"Today's Americans are still cleaning their plates, but because they've lost the ability to gauge portion sizes, they pile those plates with more food than they need.

"The unrestrained growth of portions in restaurants and in homes wouldn't be such a major concern if people simply knew when to say when," Polk continues. "Today, many Americans feel a need to polish off whatever amount of food is placed before them, even after they are full—often to the point of discomfort."

The point is simple:

We're programmed to eat all the food off our plates, no matter how crazy-big the plates get.

CHAPTER 10
ARE WE DOOMED?

THE END is NEAR

THERE IS PROBABLY NO SINGLE THING MORE OF US HAVE FAILED AT (BESIDES PROGRAMMING THE CLOCKS ON OUR VCRS AND DVD PLAYERS) THAN A DIET.

So where do we go from here? Are we doomed as a society to be overweight? I'm too optimistic a person to buy that. I've seen trends reverse and I've been part of reversing them, so I know it's possible to turn this around. Like anything, it will start small—with a few individuals who realize it's so easy once they understand the dynamics of what's happening to them and are given a tool for change. I'm a very practical person as well, and I like simple solutions that don't require a lot of thought or theory. In my mind, most diets are way too complicated and they're working against some very powerful aspects of culture.

As a result, there is probably no single thing more of us have failed at (besides programming the clocks on our VCRs and DVD players) than a diet.

The epiphany that led me to write this book was the idea that we could change our whole overstuffed, out-of-control, "super-size" food culture with one simple tool. A tool that puts everything back into perspective. It's this easy. Portions have, on average, increased by 35 to 40 percent over the past 30 years. That means calories have increased by that same amount. By going back 30 years to the smaller plate America once used, the number of calories we've

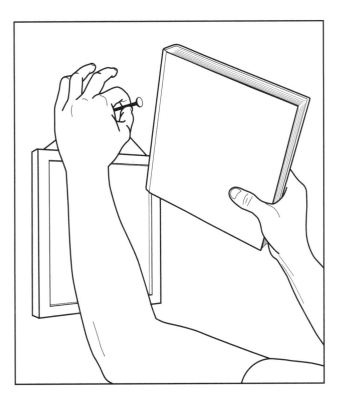

THIS BOOK IS A SIMPLE TOOL.
The nine-inch plate puts everything back into perspective.

"grown" to consume will be decreased by that same amount. Imagine cutting out all those excess calories you never wanted or needed in the first place. And imagine your senses completely convinced you're NOT on a diet.

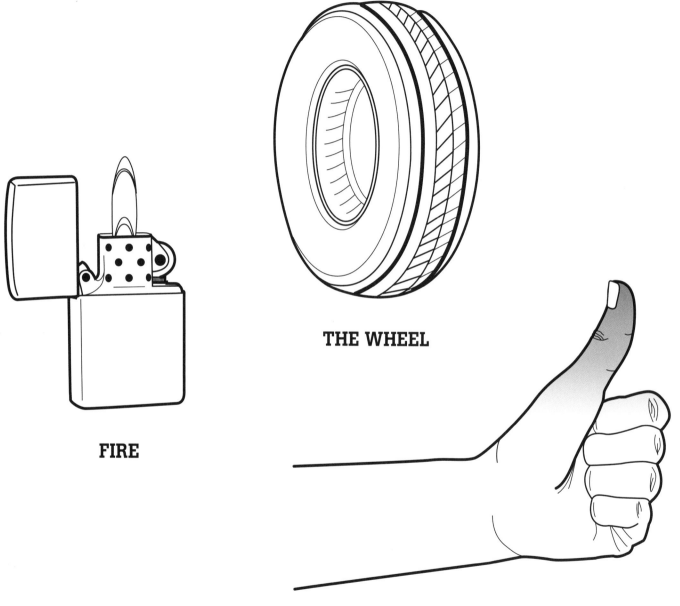

FIRE

THE WHEEL

AGRICULTURE

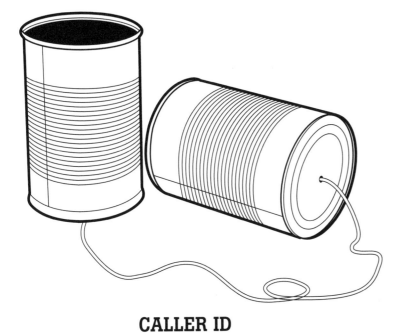

CALLER ID

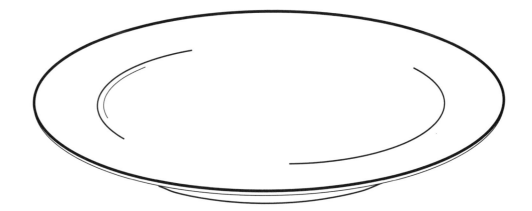

THE NINE-INCH PLATE

CHAPTER 11
WE'VE TRACED THE CALL, AND IT'S COMING FROM INSIDE THE HOUSE

Earlier, I mentioned that an important ingredient in social change is a villain to rebel against. An enemy we can keep in our minds as we make new choices. Who will it be? Where do we focus our wrath? Well, we've got no shortage of potential bad guys. From the people who sell the food to the people who package the food to the people who make the plates all the way up to the government, we have a cornucopia of villains. The problem is, I'm pretty sure none of these folks or organizations is really to blame. In a way, they're all victims. Yep, victims. Victims of the fact that their brains work in the same way yours works and mine works. That's why they make the decisions they make. Decisions that are making them fat, too.

No, they're not the real enemy. They're not the ones to be wary of. See, the whole idea of how we perceive things is what really causes all our problems. If we perceived sizes in an absolute way rather than in a relative way, we wouldn't have to worry about oversized cups, plates, or waistlines. That means the real enemy is a lot closer to home. And the real enemy is much more frightening than some Snickers brand manager who has decided to make his candy bar the size of your arm. So if this wasn't a "diet" book but was instead a horror book, right about now you'd realize the characters had made a tremendous mistake. Because the crazed psycho killer isn't outside trying to get in like we've been thinking all along. Our poor clueless victims locked all the doors and barred the windows to keep the killer out. But all they've managed to do is lock themselves in with the Jason of psychotic portions.

SO WHAT IS IT? WHAT IS THIS WEIRD, SCARY THING INSIDE US THAT FOOLS OUR EYES AND MESSES WITH OUR HEADS?

As it turns out, the source of the problem lives right downstairs in the back corner of our brain—it's called the primary visual cortex.

In a study done in 2006, neuroscientists from the University of Washington and the University of Minnesota studied the actual physiology of how we perceive images. They showed subjects a visual in which two spheres were exactly the same size, but in which one appeared larger due to the background perspective. Then, using functional magnetic resonance imaging (fMRI, to those of us who have been reading about this stuff), they examined how the brain processed the image. The spheres obviously appeared as exactly the same size on the retina, so it isn't our eyes that are fooling us. But on the primary visual cortex, which is the first part of the brain to receive signals from the eye, one sphere activated about a 20 percent larger area than the other sphere did. Stupid primary visual cortex.

Now, not surprisingly, this primary visual cortex isn't some newfangled part of the brain that just evolved in the past million years or so. It's the earliest and simplest visual area of the cortex, and it's been around roughly since mammals became mammals. It's one of the oldest and most primitive parts of our brains. And it's not all bad. It's the brain's primary processor of information about static and moving objects, it's terrific at pattern recognition, and it works its fingers to the bone by telling you where things are in relation to other things. Basically, it's really good as you run after or run away from something you want to eat or that wants to eat you. But it is a major liability at the "all you can eat" buffet. So what are you going to do, send it to its room? No. You figure out how to make it work for you instead of the other way around. Time to make the primary visual cortex into a tool of your new lifestyle. Because knowing the flaws in the primary visual cortex is going to help you create percep-

tions about what and how much you're eating—perceptions that convince your brain you're full and fulfilled without eating more food than your body needs. Basically, we're going to use the big, wrinkly, highly developed part of our brains to tame the old stupid part. We're going to learn how to be emotionally and physically satisfied.

And boy, will it feel good.

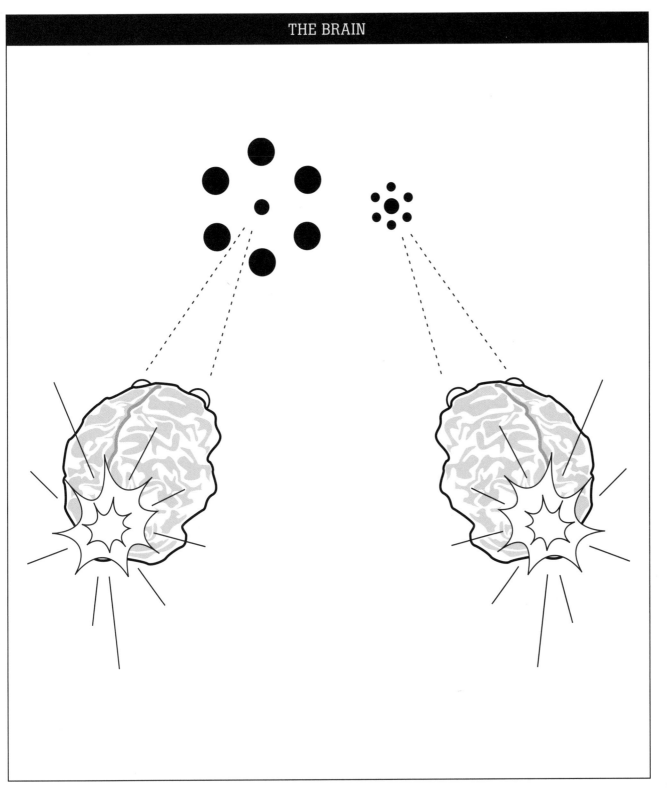

CHAPTER 12
WHAT WE'RE TALKING ABOUT
HERE IS DIET HERESY

"HEY, IT'S LOW FAT. EAT ALL YOU WANT."

"It's not what you eat but how much you eat that counts most when it comes to weight reduction," says Polk. But in a survey sponsored by the American Institute for Cancer Research, 78 percent of adults said the opposite. They believe that eating certain types of food is more important than eating less food when trying to lose weight. In the same survey, only 1 percent of the respondents could answer questions about serving sizes correctly.

How could we have it so wrong? How can we be so screwed up?

All the diets we've been exposed to have actually convinced us that what we eat is more important than how much we eat in terms of weight loss. For dozens of years, we've all been focused on types of foods and food groups. Grapefruit. Salad. Low fat. Low carb. The diets and the food industry have tried to have it both ways.

"Hey, it's low fat. Eat all you want."

And then came, "Hey, it's low carb. Eat all you want."

These famous diets all made lots of money. And Americans got lots fatter. Not that these diets are

bad; they're just really tough to stick to. As a person who is skeptical of the whole diet idea (in case you hadn't noticed), I have to admit even I was shocked at the results of a recent study done at Stanford University. Researchers there recruited 311 women who were from 15 to 100 pounds overweight and assigned each of them one of four popular diets that recommend varying amounts of carbs.

On average, over an entire year, the women lost only between three and six pounds. On the best-performing diet, which was Atkins, the women lost only an average of 10 pounds. In a year.

Now, this strikes me as a tremendous bummer and a real indictment of the industry. Not only were most of the results pretty modest, but you know those poor women were consumed every waking moment by trying to stay within the complicated requirements of the diet. And I'll bet they felt like they were starving the whole time, which is crazy because they most obviously were not starving. They lost only a few pounds over a year of torture. But their food didn't look all that satisfying on that big ol' plate, did it? And along the way, they probably cheated a little bit to make themselves feel better about that. In fact, the study admitted that people

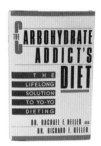

ABOVE:
This has to be stressful. You find out you're addicted to carbs but then all around you are these huge plates begging to be filled. It's like decorating an alcoholic's apartment with giant beer bottles.

"HEY, IT'S LOW CARB. EAT ALL YOU WANT."

didn't follow any of the diets to the letter. But that doesn't mean they didn't try. They did try. They tried to be successful, but the game is rigged.

Maybe now you'll understand why I decided to write a "diet" book instead of a diet book. Diet books are as culpable in this mess as the restaurants, the government, and the super-sizing movie theaters.

How can diets work in this overblown food culture? According to an American Institute for Cancer Research survey, most Americans are still unaware that the portions they consume have increased in size. Six in ten survey respondents said the portions served in restaurants are the same size or smaller, compared to ten years ago.

Eight in ten said the portions they eat at home are the same or smaller. Surprisingly, Americans under 35 years of age were more likely to recognize that their food portions had grown, compared to baby boomers and Americans 55 or older. Ironic, since these latter age groups are the very ones who grew up using nine-inch plates. Don't ask me to make sense of this one.

"Americans," Polk says, "are concentrating too exclusively on cutting fat or going on fad diets that restrict carbohydrates, sugar, or some other factor. Too often, such strategies fail to address the larger picture of total calories consumed, not to mention good nutrition."

Think about how many times diets have promised you, "Eat less and lose weight without feeling hungry," each and every one concentrating on the type of food you eat. But the secret isn't in some newfangled diet. Because no matter what you're eating, it will always be a struggle to control the amount you're eating until you know more about what makes us eat too much. What we really need to do is stop trying to fool our stomachs and learn to make our brains believe we are full and satisfied.

Let's go over that again. It's time to stop trying to fool our stomachs. And it's time to manipulate the signals to our eyes and our brains so that they help us feel satiated without overeating.

That's where your mom's old china comes in.

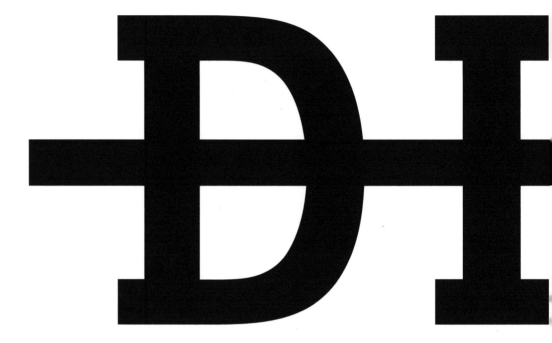

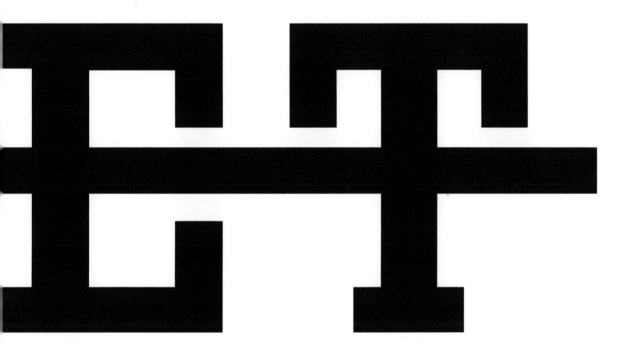

CHAPTER 13
EMOTIONAL HUNGER VS.
RATIONAL HUNGER

DID I ALREADY SAY THIS ISN'T A DIET?

You want another diet book? Check Amazon or Borders; I'm sure there's a new one coming out this week. You need to lose 10 pounds fast because your high school reunion is coming up? Jog (don't drive) to the grocery store, and buy five pounds of celery. It's the only food that actually burns up just as many calories eating it as it has in it.

The nine-inch "diet" is not about losing weight fast. It's about understanding the real dynamics that determine behavior and lead to satisfaction.

To begin with, we have to understand one more important reality about how our brains operate. When we did the truth® anti-smoking campaign, we spent a lot of time learning about how an adolescent brain actually functions. Essentially, there's a constant battle going on between the need for security and the need for independence. That, and hormones, is why most teenagers drive their parents crazy.

It's kind of the same with our brains when we're sitting down to eat.

Virtually every time you eat, you're attempting to satisfy two appetites: your rational appetite (I'll call it your ratitite) and your emotional appetite (I'll call it your emotite). If you're going out to eat in New York or LA, you may also be attempting to satisfy your publicity appetite (publitite), but that's another story.

Your ratitite is easy to understand. You burn energy when you do anything. After you've burned enough calories, your stomach growls, the "empty" light flashes, you eat to replace the calories you've burned, and you're refueled and ready to go.

The emotite has cravings that aren't so easily satisfied. Think about comfort foods. The emotite invented them. It might be great if, during times of crisis, we turned to carrot sticks and rice cakes. But not

> **RATITITE**
> –noun
> 1. a desire to satisfy a bodily need with food.

> **EMOTITE**
> –noun
> 1. a desire to satisfy an emotional craving with food.

YOU'LL BE LOOKING AT 30 TO 40 PERCENT LESS FOOD, AND YET YOU WILL BE 100 PERCENT SATISFIED.

many people have those foods at the top of their list. In general, we're talking chocolate pudding. Macaroni and cheese. Pizza. For me, it's meat loaf and mashed potatoes.

You know the Italian movies in which a family is gathered around a table heaped with pasta and meatballs and garlic bread and the grandmother is saying, "Mangia, mangia"? These are the films your emotite likes to watch.

The emotite is responsible for turning overeating into traditions—wedding cakes, Thanksgiving Day feasts, bar mitzvah buffets, Fourth of July cookouts. They were all masterminded by the emotite. The ratitite feeds the stomach. The emotite feeds the heart.

This emotional part of your brain can be a real problem. It wants one more piece of fried chicken or apple pie. It says, "I think I'll have another beer and finish up those ribs." And, when you're feeling down, it gives you the idea that six of those chocolate-covered cherries just might make you feel better. To indulge the self is how the emotite tries to help. Having a little more than you need is how you know you're taking special care of yourself. Not just with food but with anything. More pillows. More sleep. More time on vacation.

Don't get me wrong. I'm not a puritan, and I'm definitely not into self-denial. I own four motorcycles.

I know the emotite can be a very wonderful thing. It's the reason family recipes are passed down from generation to generation. It nourishes your imagination and inspires you to try new things. It's the reason that it's easier to sell a house if the kitchen smells like freshly baked bread. The trick is knowing how to use it. It may not seem like it, but you have just as much control over your emotite as your ratitite. They are both very much a part of you.

The emotite's unpredictability and ability to manipulate you are what make it a challenge. To control your emotional appetite, you have to make a plan. And how well that plan's going to work depends on how well versed you are in dealing with these two conflicting forces. It's not that the ratitite should always win over the emotite. Or vice versa. The secret is finding a balance between the two.

The nine-inch plate acts as a neutral meeting ground. The ratitite is satisfied because it's getting the amount of food it requires to stay fueled and fit. The emotite is satisfied because it perceives that it's getting plenty to eat. It must be; the plate is full. It's all about theatrics with the emotite. If it doesn't think it's missing out on anything, it's happy as a clam.

The nine-inch plate is ideal for the emotional appetite. It's been a while since the emotite has seen it, of course. Perhaps never, if you're younger than 30. But you'll be surprised how quickly the emotite adjusts to the smaller plate. Emotion is powerful, but it isn't that bright. And so, within days, you'll look down at a nine-inch plate filled with good food and you will say to yourself, "Wow, I'm not sure I can eat all that." You'll be looking at 30 to 40 percent less food, and yet you will be 100 percent satisfied.

The nine-inch plate is just the beginning, but it is the cornerstone of what will become a whole new lifestyle, and you won't even notice the change. The nine-inch plate acts as a visual reference for how much food you've consumed. Served on a dish with

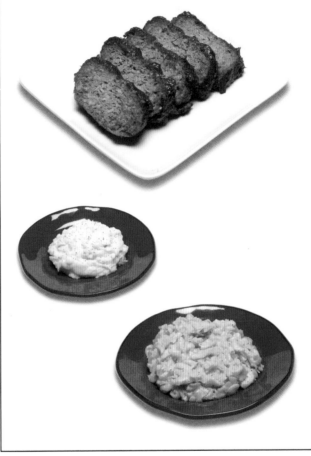

COMFORT FOODS

a nine-inch diameter, the USDA's recommended daily portions no longer look skimpy; they look just right. Now, if you're a skeptic like me, you're probably thinking, "Right, I'm going to eat 35 or 40 percent less and not notice the difference?"

All I can say is that, somehow, just about all of us as a nation used to eat 30 to 40 percent less without noticing it. If the pendulum can swing one way, it can definitely swing back the other way. Isaac Newton proved it.

CHAPTER 14
EVERYONE IN EUROPE IS ALREADY ON THIS DIET

This may come as a surprise to you (it did to me), but oversized plates are a uniquely American custom. While the standard restaurant plate in Europe is still 10 inches, the standard U.S. restaurant plate is 12 inches. And most European families use even smaller plates at home, the average being (Coincidence?) nine inches. A big reason for the smaller plate is smaller portions. They're not eating as much as we do, and it shows. Or, to be more precise, it doesn't show.

America's obesity rate is now over 30 percent. Italy and France, which a lot of people would argue have the best food in the world, have obesity rates that are less than a third of that. There are a lot of theories as to why, but we know for sure the reason isn't that they follow the latest fad diet from America (sorry, I just could not help taking another shot at diets). Overeating just isn't a part of their culture. And neither is obesity.

In his best-selling book, *The RealAge Makeover,* Dr. Michael Roizen finds, "The French—with their traditional diet heavy in fatty cheeses, butter, and red meats—had rates of cardiovascular disease that were surprisingly lower than anyone would have predicted. The hypothesis was that all the red wine the French drank to accompany their saturated-fat laden food was helping to protect their arteries from fatty plaque buildup. This hypothesis has now been modified. The French do not consume more saturated and trans fats than Americans because the French use nine-inch plates. Americans use 11- or 13-inch plates, and our portions are almost always twice the size of French portions." Wow. That was simple.

And—this is important—it's not just the plates. Although their sizes are less formalized than those of plates, the average glasses that Americans are using have ballooned just as much as our plates— maybe more.

This is a big deal. Because when it comes to calories, we drink more than anybody suspects. Our focus is always on what we're eating because that's the culture of dieting. But a huge portion of our daily caloric intake is from beverages. Some of you, no doubt, think you're way below that percentage because you drink mostly diet drinks. I'm not going to debate you here. This is not the time or place. But I will simply say this: No diet drink tastes as good as its non-diet counterpart. And if we were all drinking out of cups and glasses from circa 1950, I doubt many of us would need all these diet drinks.

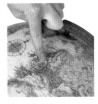

ABOVE:
Europeans seem to love trends from America. From blue jeans to hip-hop. But it looks like they took a pass on the giant-plate-big-butt thing.

FACT:
Eat off a smaller plate and you're a smaller person. Get a few million people to eat off smaller plates and you're a smaller, healthier country.

In fact, when it comes to glasses and cups, there are extremes of size that make the 30 to 40 percent plate size increase seem quite reasonable.

The classic coffee cup that served us so well for so long holds five to six ounces. The classic diner coffee cup holds eight ounces. Compare that to mugs today, which hold 10 to 12 ounces as a standard. And let's not forget the oversized decorative mugs we all love for entertaining, which can hold upwards of 16 ounces. And we'd be remiss not to mention our faithful morning companion—the travel mug—which packs a whopping 20 ounces. In the best-case scenario, we're drinking twice as much as we used to. And in some cases, we're talking about vessels that hold up to four times as much as they used to.

A coffee with cream and sugar has gone from 150 calories to 300 calories. That would be double. Simply due to the size of our glassware. To put that into some sort of extreme portion distortion perspective, in the world of plates, that would equate to a plate 18 inches across. We're talking sledding saucer.

But it's not just coffee mugs. Old-fashioned juice glasses averaged four to six ounces. Today's juice glasses come in at eight to ten ounces. And those mammoth patio glasses? They tip the scales at a massive 20 ounces!

Which reminds me of a funny story. A few years ago, we were doing the advertising for IKEA, the giant global home furnishings store. IKEA started in Sweden and became huge in Europe before coming to the U.S. When it began opening its first stores here, it struggled to adapt to how big we Americans expected everything to be. It had made stuff for most of the world for 20 years, and it all worked fine, but here people became confused by its offering. Two of the stories it told about the adjustment seemed amusing anecdotes back then, but now they take on more meaning.

In one instance, IKEA noticed it was selling a lot of chargers. A charger is the plate you sometimes see in fancy restaurants that goes under the actual plate. They're the plates we put our plates on. Nobody could understand why such a niche item was selling out constantly. And how could they be selling so many more chargers than plates? What were people putting on these chargers? Finally, with a little research, they discovered that what people were putting on them was a lot of food. Folks just thought they were buying big plates. Like the ones they were used to in restaurants.

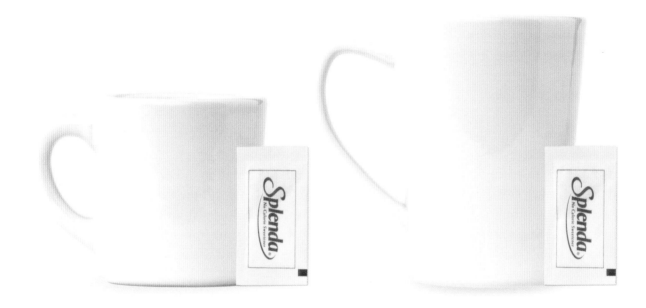

**Man is indeed a product of his environment.
As his environment gets bigger, so does man.**

As if that wasn't odd enough to these Swedes, we Americans went on to further confuse them with our love of a flower vase they made. They were having trouble keeping this one particular vase stocked. Some people were buying four, six, even eight at a time. Eventually, they discovered something that made them realize they weren't in Stockholm anymore. Their new American customers assumed IKEA's water glasses were little juice glasses and that those flower vases were something to drink soda out of. And they assumed they were buying "normal" drinking glasses when they were, in fact, buying flower vases.

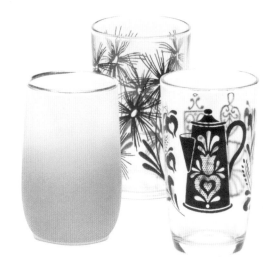

You can't make this shit up.

Polk puts it this way: "Foreigners coming to this country express amazement at the amounts of food heaped on American plates. Food adopted from foreign cuisines, such as the croissant, bagel, or quesadilla, double or triple in size when they reach our shores. Even the traditional American muffin has ballooned from a standard 1.5 ounces to as large as 8 ounces."

A team of researchers at the University of Pennsylvania and National Center for Scientific Research in Paris recently compared the size of restaurant meals and cookbook recipes in the U.S. and in France. They found that the average portion size was about 25 percent larger in America. And some were quite a bit larger than that. A candy bar sold in Philadelphia was 41 percent larger than the same product in Paris. (I'm not picking on Philadelphia; it could have been anywhere in the U.S.) They also found that the average soft drink was 52 percent larger, a hot dog was 63 percent larger, and a standard carton of yogurt was 82 percent larger.

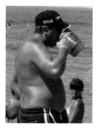

ABOVE:
Past the lips, an' over the gums… Look out, stomach! Here it comes!

Self magazine also compiled a size chart of restaurants at home and abroad. A sample of the results is on the pages that follow.

You don't have to go to Europe to see how nine-inch plates work. It's still the size of choice in a lot of American prep schools and country clubs. Even our naval officers dine from nine-inch plates, like they always have. And when's the last time you saw a fat admiral?

AND THEY ASSUMED THEY WERE BUYING "NORMAL" DRINKING GLASSES WHEN THEY WERE, IN FACT, BUYING FLOWER VASES.

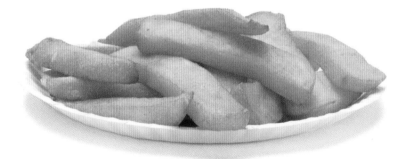

London Large Chips
5.5 Ounces, 485 Calories

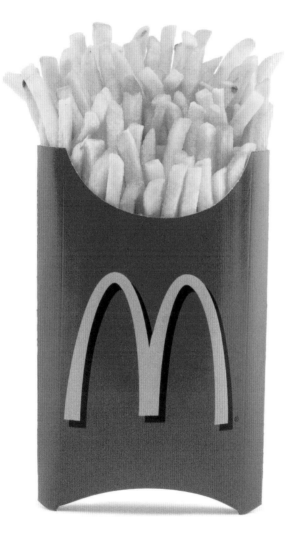

U.S. "Super-Size" Fries
7 Ounces, 610 Calories

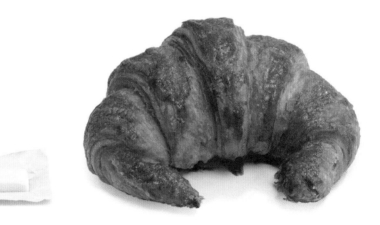

French Croissant
2 Ounces, 215 Calories

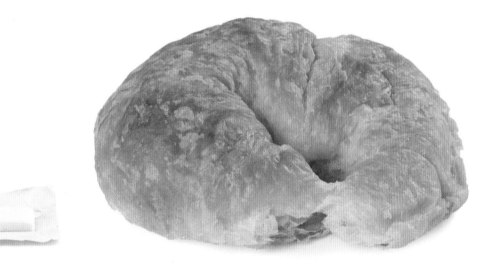

American Croissant
4 Ounces, 430 Calories

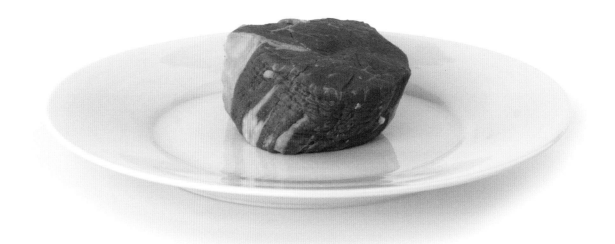

English Steak
8 Ounces, 545 Calories

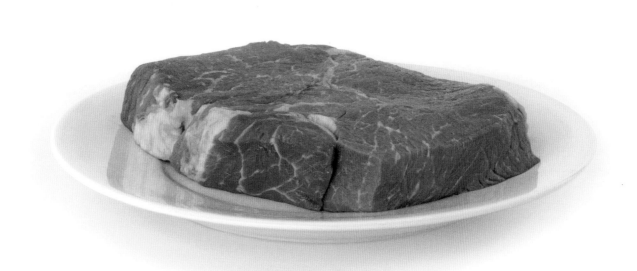

American Steak
20 Ounces, 1,360 Calories

CHAPTER 15
TOO BIG, TOO LITTLE, AND...

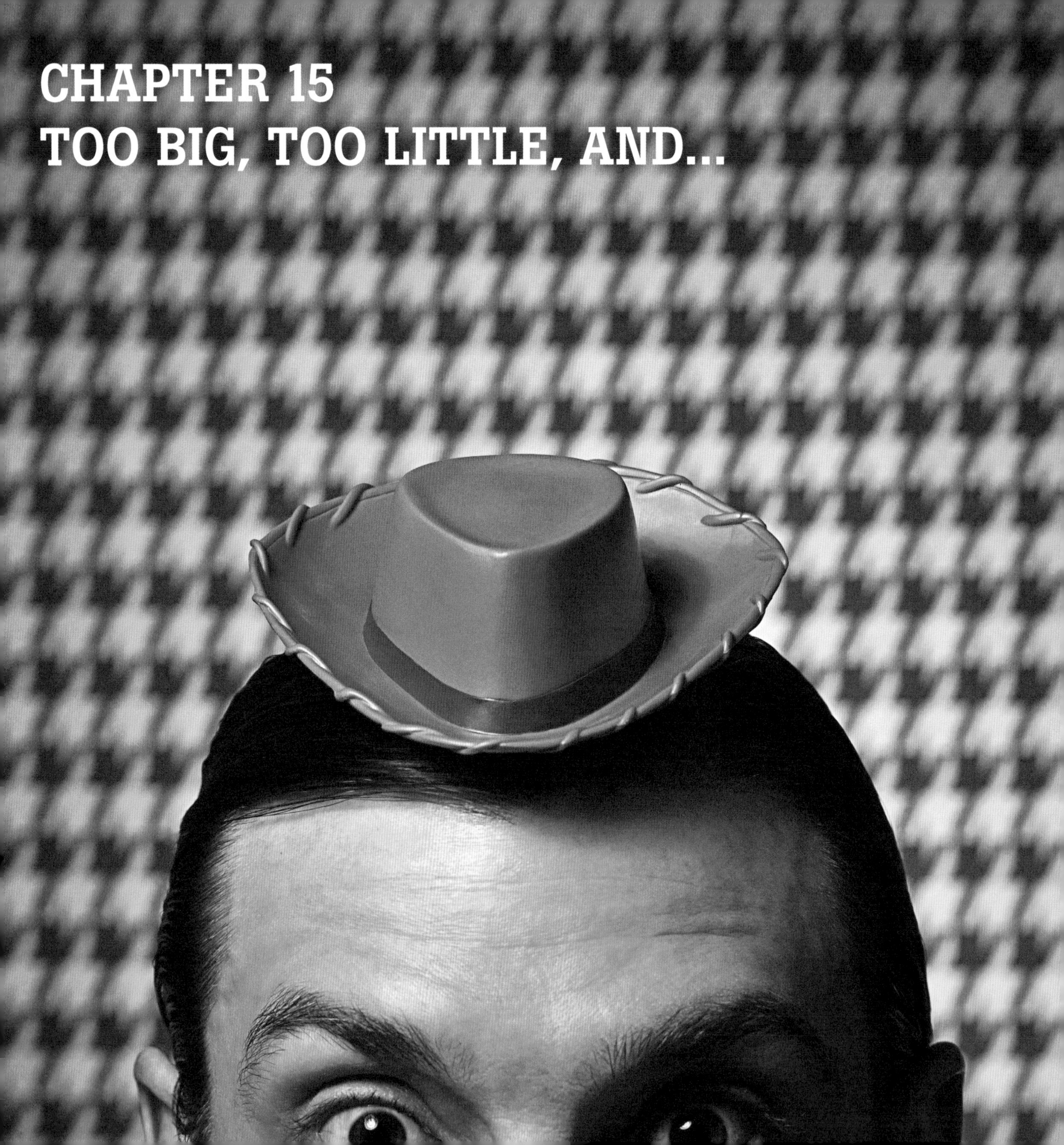

"...JUST RIGHT."

By now, you may be thinking that if a nine-inch plate is so great for losing weight and eating healthy, wouldn't an eight-inch plate be even better? See how we are? If smaller is good, then more smaller is better. Well, the answer is, probably not. Our eyes can be fooled, but they didn't just fall off a turnip truck. An eight-inch plate is a little too small for us to believe it will hold an entire dinner. Maybe that's because it won't.

A nine-inch plate has 64.53 square inches of usable space. Turns out that's just enough to hold a "normal"-size meal for a "normal"-size adult without stuff falling off the sides. People selected it because it worked better than any other size. That's probably why, for more than 100 years, the nine-inch size was the norm. Funny how things usually happen that way.

COMMIT

THE NI

PLATE A

CHANGING

TO USING

NE-INCH

ND START

YOUR LIFE.

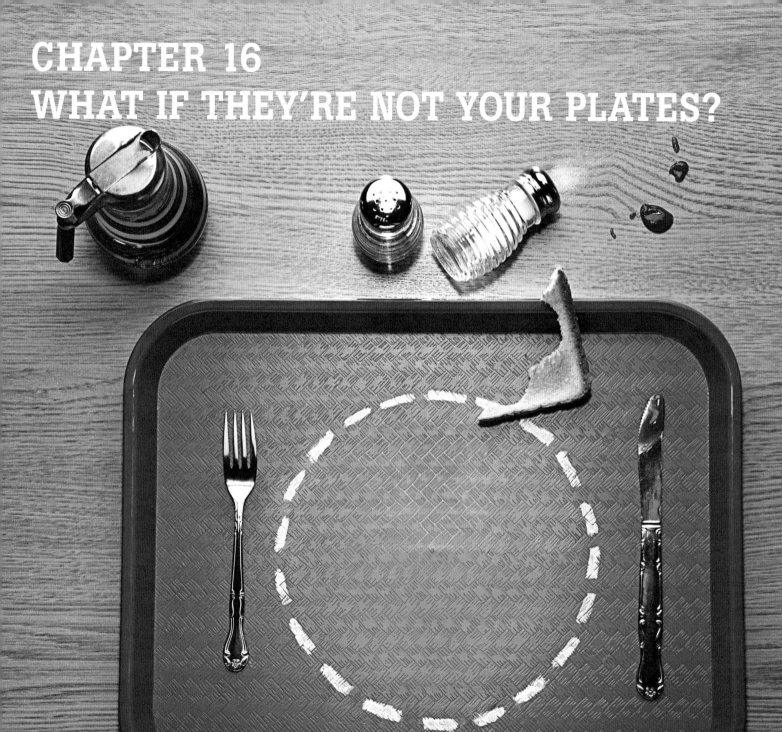

There are lots of hints and helpful advice about how to get back to a "normal," natural nine-inch plate life in the next chapter. But this problem seems to deserve a chapter of its own for one simple reason.

Americans are now eating out 30 percent of the time.

The unfortunate reality is that this idea is not going to work if you eat out all the time. It just won't. But if you eat out some of the time and take some simple steps, it will.

If you're an average American (as if there is such a thing), for just about one meal in three, you're at the mercy of somebody else's idea of how much is "enough." And since you probably won't have your nine-inch plate with you (we're working feverishly on how to solve that), your most potent weapon is a polite "no." "No. I don't want a muffin with that. No, I don't want the nine-course tasting menu. No, I don't want all the sushi I can eat. No, I don't want an even two quarts of Coke. Even if I can keep the cup."

The good news is that, as I said before, pendulums almost always work. Today, more and more restaurants are moving away from the giant-size portions of the past. It's starting, naturally, with the trendier, more expensive places, where value marketing was generally less important in the first place. The "small plate" tapas restaurants that started on the coasts are getting more popular everywhere.

Clark Wolf, a restaurant consultant in New York and San Francisco, says, "Buffets and elaborate tasting menus at upscale restaurants are passé. That's why restaurants serving small plates are so popular. You have more control over your food, but you still have the ability to cover the table and get the feeling of plenty without feeling overstuffed."

The bad news is that, aside from hedge fund managers, most of us aren't going to be eating 30 percent of our meals in multi-star restaurants. Especially with the kids.

So, here are some tips that can help. Some of them might seem a little cheesy, but they work.

FACT: If you leave it to restaurants and waiters to decide how much you should eat then you're destined to be overweight.

AMERICANS ARE NOW EATING OUT THIRTY PERCENT OF THE TIME.

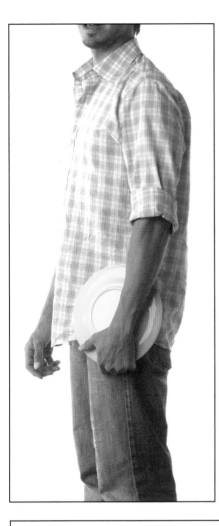

DINING OUT

Tips:

- Ask for the smallest portion they have. This may be a medium as it's become harder and harder to find small sizes on some menus.
- Check out the kids' menu. Portion size here may be more in line with a nine-inch plate. But don't bet on it.
- Use a simple mobile proxy. Spread out your fingers and flatten your hand. This is a rough equivalent to the food that fits on a nine-inch plate. Men have bigger hands on average but they also need more calories on average.
- Ask for a smaller plate. Think of the plate they gave you as a serving platter. (Helpful hint: At one time it would have been a serving platter.) Then just eat what fits on the smaller plate and doggie bag the rest so you can take it home, where portion control will be easier.
- Split main courses and desserts with a friend.
- Learn and create other methods and share those methods with others. This backlash is a work in progress and you're on the ground floor.

SEE INSIDE BACK COVER

There you will find the Handy-Dandy Portion-Control Scale-o-matic.® Otherwise known as a perforated nine-inch paper ruler.

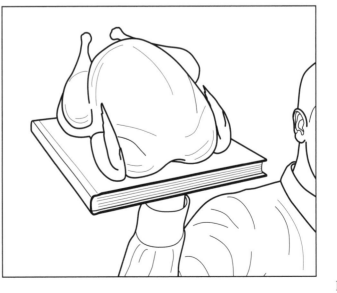

CHAPTER 17
RESTART

STEP ONE: COMMIT

STEP TWO: DUMP YOUR OLD PLATES

STEP THREE: RESTOCK YOUR CUPBOARD WITH NINE-INCH PLATES

STEP FOUR: FIND FOOD THAT FITS

STEP FIVE: DON'T ABUSE YOUR NINE-INCH PLATE

STEP SIX: END THE DIET DILEMMA

WITHIN FIVE YEARS, 95 PERCENT OF DIETERS REGAIN THEIR LOST WEIGHT.

I think I've said it three times already, but I'm going to say it again because it's probably the single most important reason why I hope this book will, in some small way, start to change the world.

Within five years, 95 percent of dieters regain their lost weight.

Why? Because they view a diet as a quick fix. And, unfortunately, that's all most fad diets are. It's why we call them "fads" instead of "legends in their own time." Don't feel bad; we've all tried one before.

Let me reiterate that. I don't hate diets. "Hate" is such an ugly word. But I like them very, very little. Because I know that Americans are fatter than ever in history and there are more diet books on the best-seller lists than ever in history.

Gosh. They don't seem to be working, do they?

What will work is if we go back to the time before Americans became overblown caricatures of themselves. To a time, not that long ago, when the best-seller lists at bookstores were about something other than carbs. Back then, the average plate size was 40 percent smaller than it is today. And it was filled with just the right amount of food.

We can go back. The nine-inch plate makes it possible. It's easy, if we take it step by step.

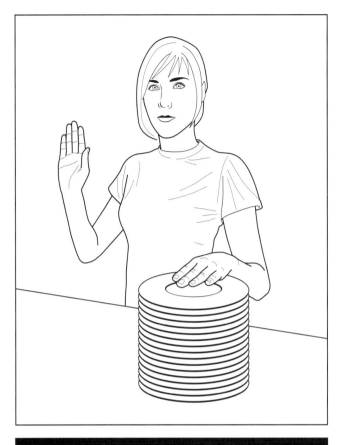

STEP ONE: COMMIT

In order to be successful, you have to look at this "diet" in a whole new way. This is not something that will run its course in two weeks. This is a lifestyle. Like brushing your teeth every day, you have to commit to using a nine-inch plate at every meal possible. Research shows it takes 30 days for new habits to form. After that, you won't even feel like you're making an extra effort. (Personally, I say screw research because I know you'll be feeling the positive effects of this "diet" in way less than a month.) Using a smaller plate will become second nature, and you won't even have to keep an eye on your portions anymore—your plate will do it for you.

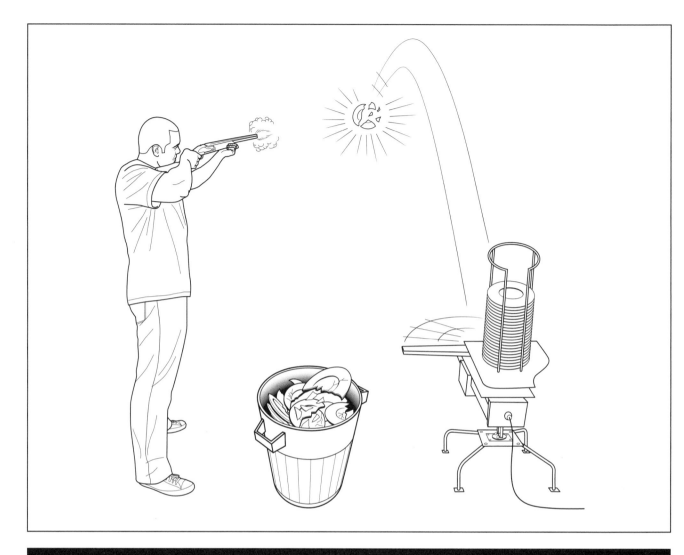

STEP TWO: DUMP YOUR OLD PLATES

Get those oversized dishes out of your cupboard. They have to go away. They have to leave the house. Even when company comes over, you need to use your nine-inch plates. It might seem embarrassing the first time, but you've learned so much already that I'll bet most of your guests will come away from dinner feeling satiated and inspired to join the revolution. Then someday, you can all laugh at how big your plates used to be. It will be fun.

So how do we get rid of the monster plates? There are lots of ways to do this. Donate them to Goodwill or the Salvation Army. Or have a garage sale. But, in a way, this feels sinister because if they're no good for you, why are they OK for other unsuspecting souls? I prefer a creative project. Paint them and make them into wall decorations. Smash them up and make a mosaic table. Or perhaps shoot skeet. Pull! You can find all kinds of creative ways to recycle your oversized dishes.

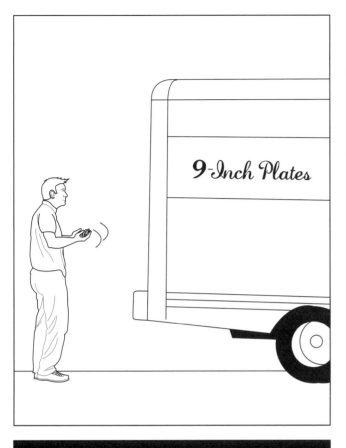

9-Inch Plates

STEP THREE: RESTOCK YOUR CUPBOARD WITH NINE-INCH PLATES

You can start this revolution today. Getting nine-inch plates at retail is getting easier and easier. I've had some luck on Amazon with Fiestaware. Also, you can find nine-inch plates (or close enough) at places like Pottery Barn, Target, and Crate and Barrel. They may label them as salad plates or dessert plates, but what do they know? Of course, any china or tableware from 1970 or earlier—when we were the appropriate size—will have plates, bowls, and cups that are the appropriate size. Wow. Another coincidence. But a page in the beginning states that the narrator doesn't believe in coincidences…. You can make it an adventure. Grab some friends, and head to your local thrift stores or flea market to select your new

china. These are some of the best outlets for your new/old dinnerware because a lot of the plates you'll find there come from the 60s and 70s. If your taste runs toward the eclectic, look for old children's plates. You can find painted Peter Rabbit scenes, or nursery rhyme motifs, or plastic plates with the Muppets or ET printed on them. You might even be able to find some old Elvis plates. Hunting on eBay can be fun, too. And you turn your new plate size hunt into a hobby and begin collecting antique table settings.

I ALREADY HAVE ENOUGH HOBBIES, IDIOT.

OK, so finding nine-inch plates can be a fun and interesting hobby. But, if I've done my job, at least some of you are thinking, "I want to do this now, right now; I want it now." (Hey, there's a bit of three-year-old in all of us.) Well, it turns out there is a way to start this diet at your next meal—just go buy some paper plates. I have to say I hesitate to even mention paper plates. I hate them. Well, not "hate," but there are few things in life I can put into a personal category of pet peeves, and paper plates and plastic utensils would have to be at the top. Go ahead and get some if you must, but please make it a short-lived, stop-gap solution. I can't bear the idea of being the cause of people's eating off paper. In addition, please be careful; these days, the "normal"-size paper plates—sorry, but we have to put "normal" in quotes again—have grown to about 10.5 inches or bigger. But all the popular paper plate makers also make smaller plates, and they're right there in the grocery store paper goods aisle. Sweetheart and Dixie both make nine-inch plates. Hefty makes an 8.875-inch plate, which is close enough, and Chinet makes a terrific heavy-duty 9-inch. All of these paper plates have the size written right on the package, plate.

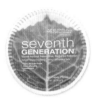

ABOVE:
Knowing that Seventh Generation plates are made from recycled paper actually makes eating off of paper feel good.

and you can buy them at every supermarket, Target, Wal-Mart, and self-respecting pharmacy in America. Bottom line, this is a really easy way to start this "diet" at your next meal. So that's good.

In fact, if you're OK eating off paper, I have a feeling you might like to take it even further. A brand called Seventh Generation makes paper plates that are made of 100 percent recycled paper and are fully biodegradable. And if you're feeling like a theme might be fun, party supply places usually have big selections of nine-inch paper and plastic plates with themes like pirate ships, poker tables, silly clowns, and *American Idol*. If you can't find them near you, go to partyadventure.com or buycostumes.com (which, by the way, has a really great nine-inch plate that looks just like a bowling ball).

I recommend when it comes to coffee cups you find some nice, classic china cups and saucers for your coffee and tea. You'll feel quite civilized, and your guests will surely be impressed with both your taste and your restraint. Or, if you feel like a more down-to-earth, casual style, get some old diner coffee cups. This stuff is easy to find. New or used. Cheap or pricey. Whatever your pleasure, you'll find it from thrift stores to restaurant supply stores to retail stores. But be careful with the new stuff. Some of what you'll find looks just like the classic stuff, but it's just slightly too outrageously inflated. It's not a bad idea to get something original on eBay or at an antique store to take with you to the store so that you have a guide.

Finally, I've included an actual-size picture of an eight-ounce glass. Remember that? It measures about five inches by 1.75 inches. And it's the perfect size for anything from water to soda. You can find these

in thrift stores, too. Warning—they're going to look stupidly small at first. But pretty soon your brain will recalibrate. You can also find these at restaurant supply companies. Either locally or online. This is an easy piece of portion control you could blow off or forget. Don't do it. The calories from beverages represent 21 percent of everything we take in. Once you start to realize that everything around you has grown, you begin to get a little paranoid. You begin to suspect bigness in items that seemed innocent enough just days earlier. That's a good sign. It may mean you're pulling yourself out of this mass state of hypnosis we all share. So what about it? What about flatware?

I can't help looking at my forks and noticing that they appear to be much larger than the forks of my childhood. They're so long that I feel like they're one step away from being effective pitchforks. A nice hunk of steak looks positively petite sitting on the ends of these babies. And the butter knife is closer to a samurai sword than what my parents buttered their toast with. That sounds like a euphemism for something naughty. "That's not how your mom and I buttered our toast, if you know what I'm saying." "Jesus, Dad, would you please not go there?" Anyway, this kind of monster knife is more comfortable with half a stick of butter hanging off it than with a pat. Not the psychological advantage we're looking for in satisfying our emotite. Nope. We gotta find some smaller utensils.

It appears as though there are three standard sizes of utensils. And it appears as though this has always been the case. Perhaps the reason I remember the smaller sizes more often than not is that, with the increase in plate sizes, more people are just opting to go with flatware that looks more proportional to the

An 8-Ounce Glass, Actual Size

plate. Huge plate. Huge flatware. It's a match made in calorie hell.

The sizes of flatware are as follows. The smallest standard size is called Place flatware. The next size up is called Dinner flatware. And the largest is called Continental flatware. Now, unless you're really not tracking with the book here, you have to realize that I recommend the Place. The great thing about it is that it's available pretty much everywhere. The bad news is you need to measure it because most retailers don't know their flatware sizes from a hole in the ground and they aren't used to people shopping by size.

STEP FOUR: FIND FOOD THAT FITS

OK, so we have a smaller plate. But with portion-growing out of control, how do we find food that fits on it? It's a little daunting when you take a look at grocery stores today. Those rectangular boxes that hold frozen TV dinners are bigger than ever before. And farmers, caught in the same gigantification wave that we all are, have injected chickens with hormones so that they produce artificially large breasts. (OK. I'm going to go right past this.) So how are we supposed to know what size is the right size? Some of us will get anal and crazy and start measuring everything, and that's cool. If you're not the type to carry your own scale, the U.S. Department of Agriculture has developed this helpful guide, estimating portion size relative to common objects. As a practical matter, though, you're going to find that your nine-inch plates are the single best tool ever invented for measuring portions. Every day, every meal, they're there to provide a simple visual clue to how much you're eating. If it looks too big on your nine-inch plate, it probably is.

There are other techniques that work. While you're at the store, ask the butcher to cut steaks in half and wrap them separately. That way, you're not putting the whole thing on the grill when you get home. Have him do the same thing with chicken breasts and whale-size fish filets. Take two seconds to take a look at labels on the products you purchase so that you really know how many portions you're eating. It's smart and doesn't take all that long to repackage foods into single-serving sizes. If a bag of cookies says that a single serving is three cookies, then put three cookies in one of those snack-size Ziploc baggies. If that seems a little obsessive to you, do it while no one's looking. If you have kids, maybe you can get them to repackage their favorite products. Get everybody in on it. It's not impossible. On the farm, when we slaughtered a pig, we didn't eat the whole thing that night.

The idea is, no one is saying you can't still shop at Costco and other warehouse clubs. After all, who can resist a lifetime supply of cheddar cheese Goldfish crackers for $10.99? Just divide the bulk container into smaller portions when you get home. In fact, seeing bulk containers for what they are is a good exercise in understanding rational portions.

STEP FIVE: DON'T ABUSE YOUR NINE-INCH PLATE

I'm not going to tell you exactly what to eat; just use common sense when filling your plate.

Two of these examples illustrate the wrong way to use your nine-inch plate. Can you guess which one is right?

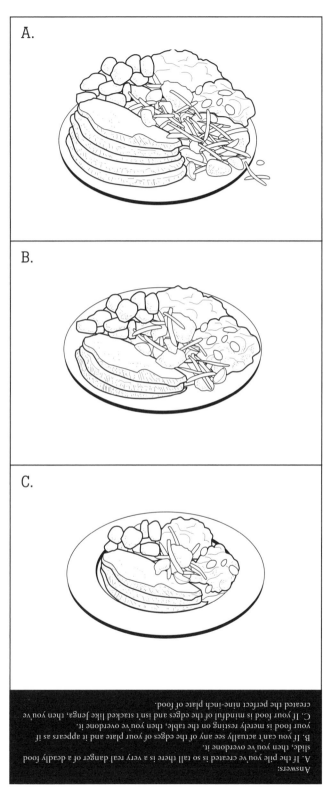

A.

B.

C.

Answers:
A. If the pile you've created is so tall there is a very real danger of a deadly food slide, then you've overdone it.
B. If you can't actually see any of the edges of your plate and it appears as if your food is merely resting on the table, then you've overdone it.
C. If your food is mindful of the edges and isn't stacked like Jenga, then you've created the perfect nine-inch plate of food.

STEP SIX: END THE DIET DILEMMA

So the person you live with is not a "diet" person. That doesn't mean you can't both benefit from using nine-inch plates. So often, diets fail because they draw a line between two people. You can't go out to your favorite Italian restaurant because he can't have carbs. Or you won't eat the birthday cake she made you because you're on Sugar Busters. One way of eating invariably alienates the other. The nine-inch plate is your common ground. The great equalizer. You may be on the Atkins diet, but that doesn't mean your partner can't enjoy a slice of pizza. Just be sure to serve both meals on nine-inch plates.

You may try different diets throughout your life, but when you're using the nine-inch plate, your approach to eating whichever type of food that diet recommends doesn't need to change.

Look, I don't love most diets (for the 50th time), but I'm not completely naïve either. I know that sometimes we all decide to go on some sort of low carb diet to try to get ready for our high school reunion or to squeeze into an ugly bridesmaid dress. Cool. And guess what? The perfect time to start the nine-inch "diet" is before you start another diet. Because then, after you dump your fad diet like a hot potato, you'll be in the perfect position to keep the weight off that you meant to lose in the first place. Your lifestyle will keep the weight off and slowly and painlessly ease you down to your natural weight.

CHAPTER 18
NINE-INCH VERSIONS OF YOUR FAVORITE DIETS

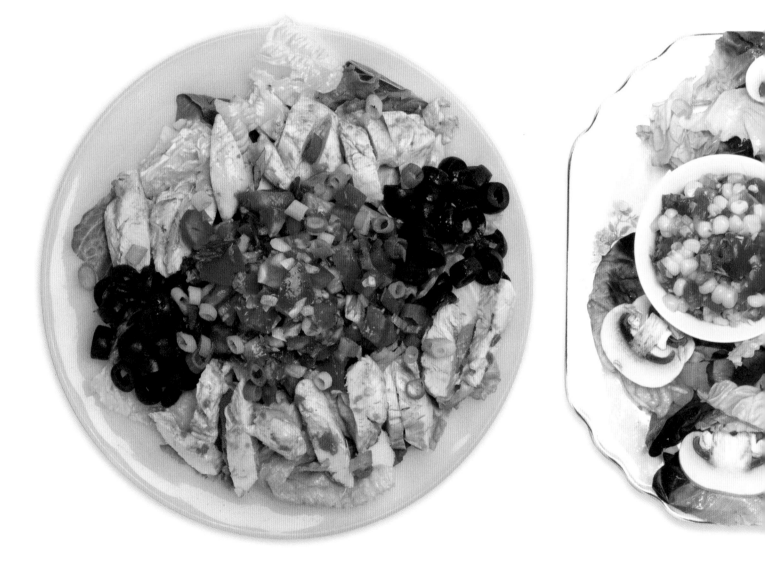

The Personality Type Diet

Su

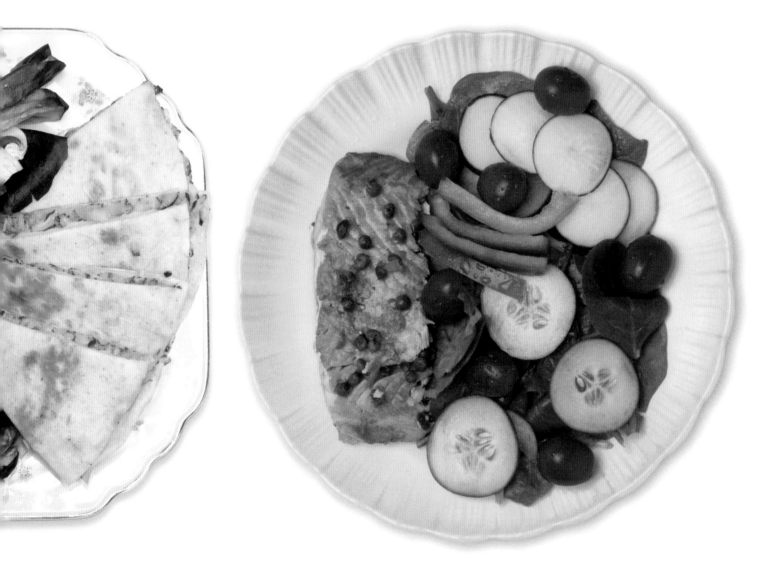

sters!

What Color Is Your Diet?

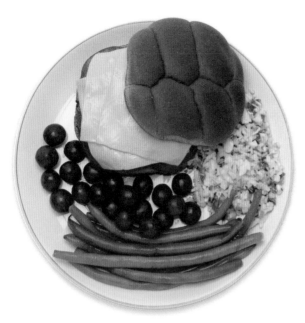

The Pritikin Principle

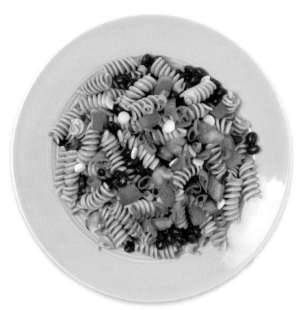

Weight Watchers

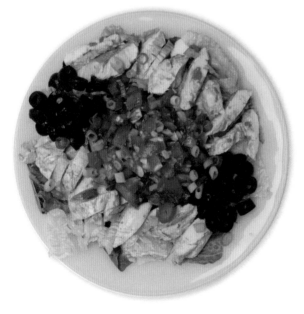

Living Low Carb

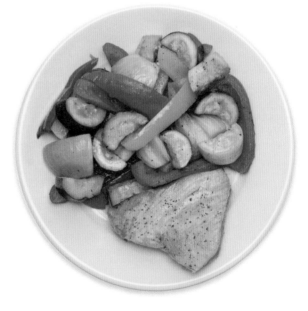

The Slim-Fast Plan

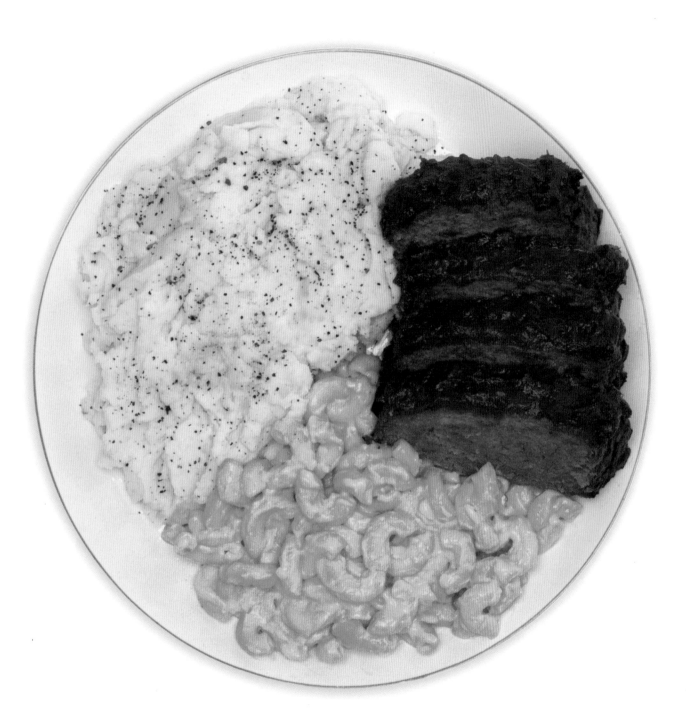

The Atkins Diet

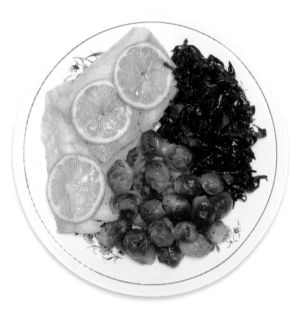

The Fat Fallacy

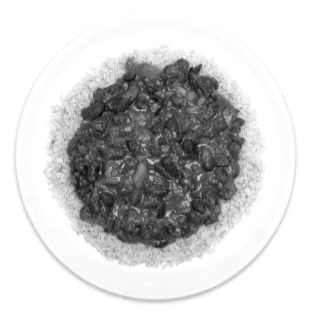

Volumetrics

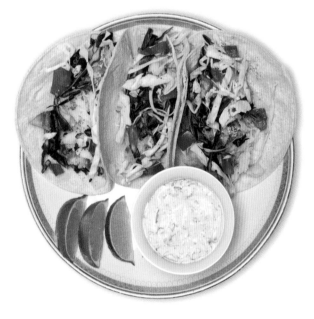

The South Beach Diet

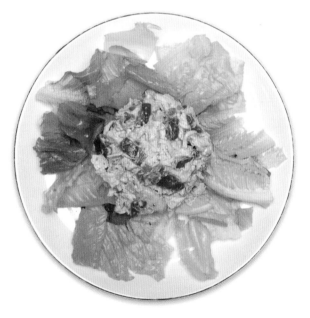

The Ornish Diet

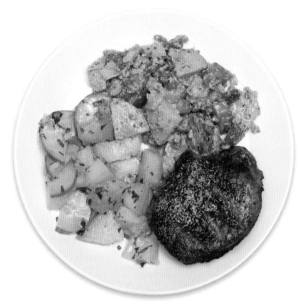

The RealAge Makeover

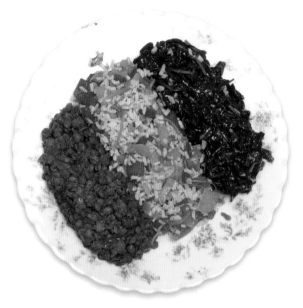

Body-for-LIFE

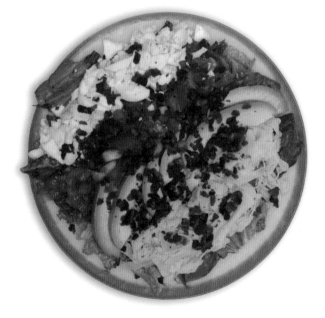

The Zone Diet

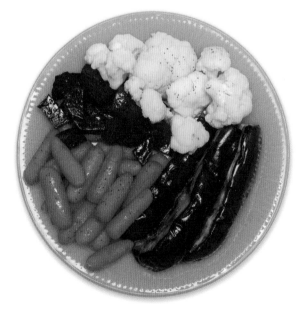

The Carbohydrate Addict's Diet

THE TOKEN RECIPE:
MEAT LOAF

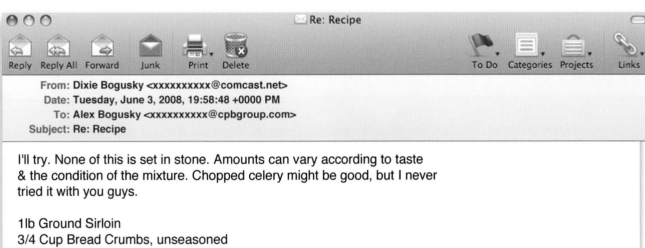

Reply Reply All Forward   Junk   Print   Delete   To Do   Categories Projects   Links

From: **Dixie Bogusky <xxxxxxxxxx@comcast.net>**
Date: **Tuesday, June 3, 2008, 19:58:48 +0000 PM**
To: **Alex Bogusky <xxxxxxxxxx@cpbgroup.com>**
Subject: **Re: Recipe**

I'll try. None of this is set in stone. Amounts can vary according to taste
& the condition of the mixture. Chopped celery might be good, but I never
tried it with you guys.

1lb Ground Sirloin
3/4 Cup Bread Crumbs, unseasoned
1-2 Eggs
Chopped Onion (optional)
Salt, pepper, seasoning to taste

Mix well, form a loaf, top with ketchup.
Bake at 350 degrees until done (45-60 min.)
Serves 6-8

-------------- Original message ----------------------

From: Alex Bogusky <xxxxxxxxxx@cpbgroup.com>
Date: Tue, 03 Jun 2008 19:32:158 +0000
To: Dixie Bogusky <xxxxxxxxxx@comcast.net>
Subject: Recipe

Mom,

Will you send me that meat loaf recipe again?

Love,
Alex

CHAPTER 19
SPREAD THE NINE-INCH PLATE LOVE

WILLPOWER IS A MYTH

We all love stories of willpower. Stories of people who knew what they needed to do and just did it. Even though every ounce of their body was telling them to do something else. Many of these tales come from smokers. Smokers who didn't need a patch or hypnosis to drop the habit. Well, from my work in this area, I can tell you there are people who just quit smoking without any help. But the idea that the difference was some sort of inner strength is complete baloney. And it's baloney of the most destructive kind because it makes people who can't quit feel like there's something wrong with them. The reality is that in the "normal" pattern, it takes seven attempts to successfully quit. The addiction is that serious. And the reason is this: There are receptors in the brain that accept the nicotine. But unlike most drugs, nicotine actually stimulates the brain to grow more receptors. So a person's brain essentially rewires itself to work better with nicotine. This happens 90 percent of the time. Yet for some reason, there are some people who never grow these additional receptors. And so for them, quitting smoking after years of the habit is not much harder than if they had decided to quit after the first cigarette they ever smoked. They were never really addicted to nicotine. Just to the habit.

The point is, most of us aren't addicted to food. We're caught up in the habit of eating too much because "too much" has been the portion in front of us for a long time. So screw willpower. Screw feeling hungry. Screw being obsessed with a diet every moment of every day. Behavioral research says it's going to take you a month or so to get used to eating off nine-inch plates. I say the sooner you forget about it, the better. Earlier in the book, as I was going on about diets, I cited that with Atkins, the average person lost 10 pounds over a year. With the next-best diet, people lost less than half that. Four pounds. What pains me is that I know that those people spent every waking moment obsessing over food and their diet for a year for a measly four pounds. My goodness. We don't need that. That's not going to make anybody happy. Losing weight should feel just like putting on weight. It should happen without too much thought. So put all your plans in place for your nine-inch "diet," and then just kick into living better. You won't want to eat any other way. And why not?

What you'll have discovered is an uncomplicated way to get back to the "you" that you were supposed to be in the first place—or that you used to be.

You'll have done, perhaps, the biggest favor you could ever do for yourself. And who knows? You may want to do the same for others. I know that's been my instinct since I started writing the book. I've been turning anybody that will listen on to what I've learned. You've found a lifestyle that will help you maintain your weight and health for years and years to come. So it only makes sense that you'd want your friends and family—especially your kids—to reap the same benefits.

So, if you start to get the same feeling, then share this book with them after you've finished reading it. The reality is that it's not a completely selfless act. If you have friends, or in my case parents, who have you over for dinner a lot, you're going to want to convert them to make life a little easier for you, too. Maybe lead by example. Invite friends over for a dinner party to break in your new nine-inch plates. (Going to their house? A set of four makes a lovely hostess gift.) Who knows? If enough people join this cupboard crusade, we might even end up reversing America's seemingly unstoppable trend toward the gigantic. In a couple of years, the nine-inch plate could become standard restaurant-ware again. With all that extra room on the table, we'd be able to invite another friend to dinner.

Maybe after 40 years, our food culture will be completely reformed. And somebody will stumble across a copy of this book and wonder, "What kind of idiot would write a diet book about nine-inch plates? All plates are nine inches." Now, that would be cool.

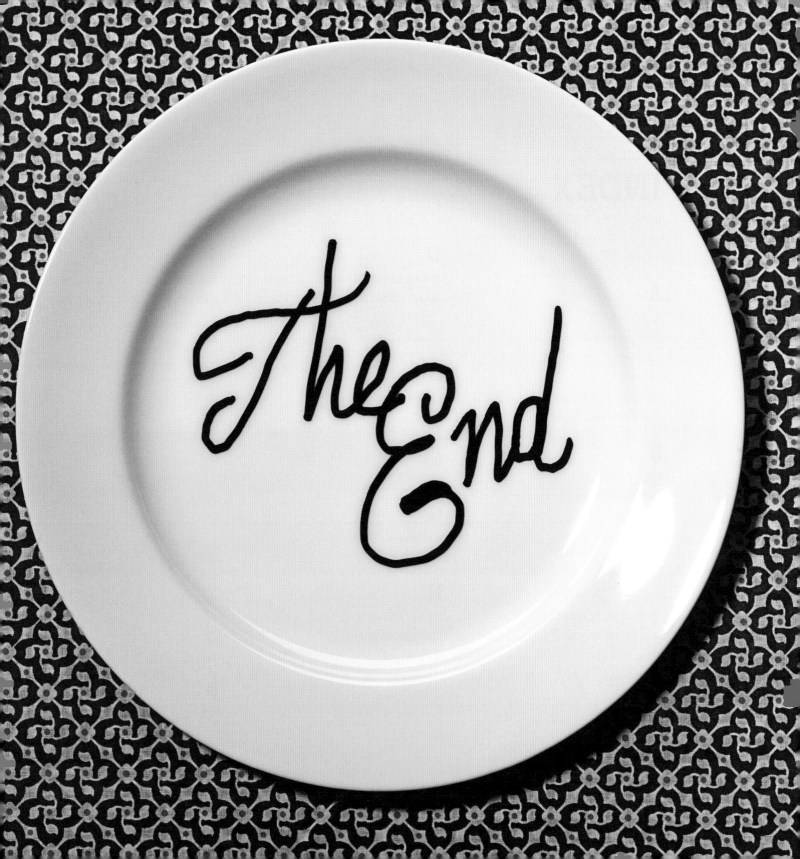

INDEX

CONTRIBUTORS

DESIGN
Paul Sahre

ART DIRECTION
Mike Kohlbecker
David Steinke
Jason Ambrose
Mel Kreilein

PHOTOGRAPHY
Adam Fish of Fish Fotography
David Mejias
Melissa Melendez

PHOTO STYLING
Molly Terry
Miranda Parker

RETOUCHING
Mark Ross Studio
Michael Flynn
Casey Kerrick

ILLUSTRATION
James Victore
Andrew Dixon
Joshua Merced
Wayne Porter

The 9-Inch "Diet"

© 2008 powerHouse Cultural Entertainment, Inc.
Text © 2008 Alex Bogusky and Chuck Porter
Illustrations © 2008 James Victore, Andrew Dixon,
Joshua Merced, and Wayne Porter

Published in the United States by powerHouse Books,
a division of powerHouse Cultural Entertainment, Inc.
37 Main Street, Brooklyn, NY 11201-1021
telephone 212 604 9074, fax 212 366 5247
e-mail: 9inchdiet@powerHouseBooks.com
website: www.powerHouseBooks.com

First edition, 2008

Library of Congress Cataloging-in-Publication Data:

Bogusky, A. M. (Alex M.)
  The 9-inch diet : exposing the big conspiracy in America / by Alex
Bogusky; with a little help from Chuck Porter.
      p. cm.
  ISBN 978-1-57687-320-5 (hardcover)
  1. Reducing diets. 2. Weight loss. I. Porter, Chuck. II. Title.

  RM222.2.B5897 2009
  613.2'5--dc22

                              2008037364
Hardcover ISBN 978-1-57687-320-5

Printing and binding by Oceanic Graphic Printing, Inc., China
Book design by Paul Sahre

A complete catalog of powerHouse Books and Limited Editions is
available upon request; please call, write, or visit our website.

10 9 8 7 6 5 4 3 2 1

Printed and bound in China